Elizabeth Cook

RENAL DIET

The Definitive Guide to Manage This Disease.
How to Improve the Renal Function and
How to Avoid Dialysis.
What to Eat and Not, Daily Quantities to
Get Potassium, Phosphorus, Fluid, and Sodium

© Copyright 2020 - All rights reserved.

The content contained within this book may not be reproduced, duplicated or transmitted without direct written permission from the author or the publisher. Under no circumstances will any blame or legal responsibility be held against the publisher, or author, for any damages, reparation, or monetary loss due to the information contained within this book. Either directly or indirectly.

Legal Notice:

This book is copyright protected. This book is only for personal use. You cannot amend, distribute, sell, use, quote or paraphrase any part, or the content within this book, without the consent of the author or publisher.

Disclaimer Notice:

Please note the information contained within this document is for educational and entertainment purposes only. All effort has been executed to present accurate, up to date, and reliable, complete information. No warranties of any kind are declared or implied. Readers acknowledge that the author is not engaging in the rendering of legal, financial, medical or professional advice. The content within this book has been derived from various sources. Please consult a licensed professional before attempting any techniques outlined in this book.

By reading this document, the reader agrees that under no circumstances is the author responsible for any losses, direct or indirect, which are incurred as a result of the use of information contained within this document, including, but not limited to, errors, omissions, or inaccuracies.

Table of Contents

INTRODUCTION 4

CHAPTER ONE: UNDERSTANDING HOW THE KIDNEY FUNCTIONS 6
- Kidney Anatomy 6
- Kidney Functions 7
- Additional Information 8

CHAPTER TWO: UNDERSTANDING KIDNEY DISEASE 9
- Stages of Chronic Kidney Failure 10
- Kidney Diseases—Causes, Symptoms, Diagnosis, and Treatment 14

CHAPTER THREE: BENEFITS OF FOLLOWING A RENAL DIET 17
- Why Is It So Important to Follow a Meal Plan? 17
- Fundamentals of the Renal Diet 18
- What Is the Difference Between Kidney Diets? 23
- Special Dietary Concerns 26

CHAPTER FOUR: HOW TO IMPROVE KIDNEY FUNCTION 28
- Eat Healthily 28
- Drink Healthily 29
- Weight Control and Regular Exercise 30
- The Emergence of Kidney Disease 31
- How to Avoid Dialysis 32
- Steps to Control Chronic Kidney Failure 33

CHAPTER FIVE: FOODS TO AVOID IF YOU HAVE BAD KIDNEY 36
- Cola Soda 37
- Avocados 38
- Canned Food 39
- Wholemeal Bread 40
- Integral Rice 41
- Bananas 42
- Dairy Products 42
- Oranges and Orange Juice 44
- Processed Meats 45
- Pickles, Olives, and Sauce 45
- Apricots 46
- Potatoes and Sweet Potatoes 47
- Tomatoes 48
- Packaged, Instant, and Prepared Meals 48
- Swiss Chard, Spinach, and Beet Greens 49

- Dates, Raisins, and Plums 50
- Pretzels, Chips, and Cookies 51
- Best Foods for People with Kidney Disease 52
- Daily Tips to Boost Your Kidney Function 61

CHAPTER SIX: DIET FOR CHRONIC KIDNEY DISEASE 62

- High-Calorie Intake 62
- Protein Restriction 64
- Water intake 64
- Helpful Tips to Reduce Water Intake 66
- Salt Restriction (Sodium) 68
- Practical Advice to Reduce Your Salt Intake 70
- Potassium Restriction 71
- The Restrictive Phosphorus Diet 75
- Designing a Daily Diet 76

CHAPTER SEVEN: 7-DAY PLAN: WHAT TO EAT TO DETOXIFY YOUR KIDNEYS FAST 79

- Kidneys Detox Day 1 80
- Kidneys Clean Day 2 81
- Kidneys Clean Day 3 81
- Kidneys Clean Day 4 82
- Kidneys Clean Day 5 83
- Kidneys Clean Day 6 84
- Kidneys Clean Day 7 84
- Myths and Facts about Kidney Disease 85

Introduction

The kidney is a wonderful organ that is important to your body's health through waste the elimination and excretion. Although the primary function of a kidney is the purifying function, the kidneys play a major role in regulating the blood pressure, fluid volume, and electrical concentrations in the body.

However, nearly everyone has two kidneys at birth, but in the last few years, the human body can function with only one kidney, increasing in patients with diabetes and highly bloated pain. It enables us to help people to become aware of this plague and to explain diseases better.

This book will be about kidneys, disease prevention, and the value of early treatment. The aim is to help patients better understand and manage the disease of the kidneys when it occurs.

If you experience chronic diseases such as high blood pressure, diabetes, heart and kidney disease, what you eat is crucial. Patients suffering from chronic kidney disease normally have a diet tailored by their doctor. This diet will continue to change constantly, depending on the state of the renal disease. Be sure that you keep a journal of what you eat every day as a patient with renal disease. This is essential for your nutritionist. It is also important to invest in a scale every morning to monitor your weight. In most cases, individuals with chronic kidney disease have to gain weight or retain weight.

If you lose too much bodyweight, your dietician may add extra calories to your diet. When you eat more calories than your body spends, you get a weight gain. That is why most people are obese and overweight. On the other hand, your dietician can guide you safely to reduce your daily calorie intake and increase your activity if you gain too much weight. Additional operations consume the energy of the mire. It is a matter of concern that you can quickly gain weight, as it may be a sign that your body has too much fluid. Doctors specifically seek weight gain along with swelling, shortness of breath, and increased blood pressure.

For your overall condition and feeling, when you have chronic kidney disease, it is important to get the right amount of protein. When building muscles, repairing tissues and fighting infections, your body needs the right amount of protein. If your protein levels are not adequate, you may be advised by your doctor to use a diet that has a controlled amount of protein.

This reduces the amount of waste in your blood and may make your kidneys work longer. Protein can be taken individually from two sources, namely plant and animal sources. Animal sources include eggs, fish, chicken, red meat, milk and cheese. Plants are also included in vegetables and grains.

Besides protein, you need to have other significant nutrients in your diet. Nutrients are available that you need in the right amount to be in your best daily condition. Sodium is one of these. A combination of kidney, high blood pressure, and sodium is often found. It is important to limit sodium in your diet to keep your blood pressure under control. Control of your high blood pressure is of primary importance when you suffer from kidney disease. This means eating fewer salt foods or salt alternatives.

Chapter One:
Understanding How the Kidney Functions

The balance of the internal chemistry of our bodies is largely due to the kidneys' work. Our survival depends on these vital organs functioning normally.

The kidneys are responsible for four functions in the body:

- Elimination of toxins from the blood by a filtration system;
- Regulation of blood and bone formation;
- Blood pressure regulation;
- Control of the delicate chemical and liquid balance of the body.

The kidneys are vital organs, as essential to our life as our heart or our lungs. However, they remain poorly understood, just like the diseases that affect them.

These so-called silent diseases are, in a good number of cases, diagnosed too late, while early and appropriate management can slow or even stop their development.

When faced with kidney failure and its treatments, getting informed and understanding is essential.

Kidney Anatomy

Each person normally has two kidneys, but one kidney is enough to live.

The kidneys are flattened, ovoid, and complex functioning organs.

Contrary to popular belief that the kidneys are located in the lower back, they are located just below the rib cage (at the last ribs' height).

Kidney Functions

The Main Purpose of the Kidneys

The main function of the kidneys is to remove water and water-soluble substances (end products of metabolism) from the body. The excretory function is closely related to the regulation function of the ionic and acid-base balance of the internal environment of the body. Hormones control both functions. Also, the kidneys perform an endocrine function, taking a direct part in synthesizing many hormones. Finally, the kidneys are involved in intermediate metabolic processes, especially in gluconeogenesis and cleavage of peptides and amino acids.

A very large volume of blood passes through the kidneys: 1500 litres per day. From this volume, 180l of primary urine is filtered. Then the volume of primary urine is significantly reduced due to the reabsorption of water; thus, the daily output of urine is 0.5–2.0 litres.

Process of Urination

The kidney's functional (and structural) unit is the nephron; there are approximately 1 million nephrons in the human kidney. The nephrotic urination process consists of three phases:

- **Ultrafiltration (glomerular or glomerular filtration).** In the glomeruli of the renal corpuscles, primary urine is formed from blood plasma during ultrafiltration, isosmotic with blood plasma. The pores through which the plasma is filtered have an effective average diameter of 2.9nm. With this pore size, all blood plasma components with a molecular weight up to 5 kDa freely pass through the membrane. Substances with M <65 kDa partially pass through the pores, and only large molecules (M> 65 kDa) are retained by the pores and do not enter the primary urine. Since most blood plasma proteins have a fairly high molecular weight (M> 54 kDa) and are negatively charged; they are retained by the glomerular basement membrane. The protein content in the ultrafiltration is insignificant.

- **Reabsorption.** Primary urine is concentrated (about 100 times the original volume) due to the reverse filtration of water. At the same time, by the mechanism of active transport, practically all low-molecular substances, especially glucose, amino acids, as well as most electrolytes (inorganic and organic ions) are reabsorbed in the tubules. The reabsorption of amino acids is carried out using group-specific transport systems (carriers), with a defect associated with several genetically determined hereditary diseases (cystinosis, glycosuria, Hartnup's syndrome).

Additional Information

- **Metabolism.** Concentration and selective transport processes are energy-intensive. The required ATP is synthesized through the oxidation of fatty acids, ketone bodies, and some amino acids, and to a lesser, extent lactate, glycerol, citrate, and glucose, which are found in the blood. In the kidneys, just like in the liver, the process of gluconeogenesis can take place. The substrates are the carbon skeletons of glucogenic amino acids, the nitrogen of which ammonia is used to regulate urine pH. In the kidneys, enzymes of the cleavage of peptides and amino acids' metabolism are found with high activity (for example, amino acid oxidase, amine oxidase, and glutaminase).

- **Renal clearance (renal cleansing).** This is the most used indicator by which the rate of renal excretion of certain substances from the blood is determined. It is defined as the volume of blood plasma purified from a specific substance per unit of time. The clearance of inulin, polyfructazan with $M \approx 6kDa$, which is well filtered, but does not undergo active reabsorption and secretion, serves as an indicator of the glomerular filtration rate. The normal value of the glomerular filtration rate, determined by inulin, is 120ml/min.

Chapter Two:
Understanding Kidney Disease

Only in the United States, kidney conditions are estimated to affect 31 million people, and at a worldwide level, one of each ten people has a kidney disease. Kidney disease, also known as renal disease, is the overall term for damage, reducing kidney function. Chronic kidney disease (CKD) occurs when the kidneys can no longer clear and function with toxins and wastes from the blood. This can happen suddenly or overtime. There are five different phases of chronic kidney disease (CKD).

Our two kidneys every day philtre approximately 120 to 150 quarters of kidney blood and produce approximately 1 to 2 quarts of waste urine and extra fluid.2 Healthy kidneys help regulate blood pressure, remove rubbish and water, signal that your body is making red blood cells and help control childhood growth.

The chronic renal failure or uremia is the kidneys' inability to produce urine or fabricate low quality ("like water") since it has not been removed enough toxic waste. Although some patients continue to urinate, most cannot. However, the important thing is not the quantity, but the composition or quality of the urine.

The kidneys are two "bean-shaped" organs located in the dorsal wall of the body on the sides of the spine. They are brown, weigh about 150-grams each, and are about 12 centimetres long, 6 centimetres wide, and 3 centimetres thick. In the upper part, each kidney has an endocrine gland attached (it produces vital substances inside the body) called the adrenal gland.

The kidneys are the "purifiers" where the blood is filtered and cleaned. They produce urine, which contains water, toxins, and salts that the blood has been collecting throughout the body, and that has to be eliminated. They also intervene in other activities such as reproduction because they make sex hormones; regulate the amount of phosphorus and calcium in the bones; they control the tension in the blood vessels, and manufacture substances involved in blood clotting.

Renal insufficiency appears when only 5 per cent of the total kidney or nephron filters work. The basic unit of the kidney is the nephron, of which there are about 1 million in each organ. Each nephron is formed by a component that acts as a filter, the glomerulus, and a transport system, the tubule.

Some of the blood that reaches the kidneys is filtered by the glomerulus and passes through the tubules. Various excretion and reabsorption processes occur, resulting in urine that is eventually removed.

The renal blood flow (RBF or amount of blood reaching the kidney per minute) is approximately 1.1 litres per minute in adults. Of the 0.6 litres of plasma that enter the glomerulus through the arterioles, 20 per cent are filtered, an operation called renal glomerular filtration.

The renal glomerular filtrate is, therefore, the volume of plasma filtered by the kidneys per unit of time. The amount of filtered plasma per day is 135 to 160 litres. To prevent fluid loss, between 98 per cent and 99 per cent of the renal glomerular filtration rate is reabsorbed by the tubules, resulting in the amount of urine removed resulting from between one and two litres per day.

When a kidney disorder occurs, it means that one or more of the renal functions are altered. But not all functions are altered in the same proportion; if, for example, two-thirds of the nephrons cease to function, significant changes may not occur because the remaining nephrons adapt. Likewise, changes in hormonal production may go unnoticed, and then the calculation of renal glomerular filtration is the only way to detect the decrease in the number of nephrons that continue to function.

Stages of Chronic Kidney Failure

An average of 180 litres of blood per day is filtered by the two kidneys, about 90 to 125ml per minute. The rate of glomerular filtration or creatinine clearance is called this.

The phases of chronic renal failure are divided by the rate of glomerular filtration, which can be estimated using creatinine levels in the blood. To estimate the degree of functioning of the kidneys from the values of creatinine, several mathematical formulas exist. Nowadays, when creatinine dosage is requested, most laboratories already automatically do this calculation.

Renal failure, with a deterioration of function over the years, is often a progressive illness. The risk of rapid kidney function loss is increased by certain factors, such as poorly controlled diabetes and hypertension.

We have divided the IRC stages as follows:

CKD Stage 1

Patients with creatinine clearance greater than 90 ml/min but any of the above-described diseases (diabetes mellitus, high blood pressure, polycystic kidneys, etc.)

Patients with one or more of these conditions always have some degree of kidney damage that, however, may not yet be reflected in the blood's filtering capacity. They are patients with normal renal function, with no symptoms, but a high risk of deterioration of long-term renal function.

With normal creatinine, but with changes in the urine test, patients also reach this stage, with signs of bleeding or protein loss in the urine.

Stage 2

Patients with creatinine clearance between 60 and 89 ml/min.

This can be called the pre-renal failure stage. They are people with small losses of kidney function, being the earliest stage of kidney failure.

As the kidneys lose function naturally with age, many older people may have slightly reduced kidney function. This drop-in function is simply a sign of the ageing of the kidneys. Therefore, finding older people with criteria for stage II CRF is extremely common. If the patient does not have any disease that attacks the kidneys, such as diabetes or hypertension, this slight kidney function loss does not cause major problems in the medium/long term.

In stage II, the kidney is still able to maintain its basic functions, and blood creatinine is still very close to the normal range. However, it is important to note that these patients are at greater risk of worsening renal function if exposed, for example, to drugs that are toxic to the kidneys, such as anti-inflammatory drugs or contrasts for radiological examinations.

Stage 3

Patients with creatinine clearance between 30 and 59 ml/min.

This is the stage of chronic renal failure that has been declared. Creatinine is already higher than the reference values, and the first disease complications are beginning to develop. The kidney has already decreased its ability to produce erythropoietin, a hormone that controls bone marrow production of red blood cells, causing the patient to develop progressive anaemia.

Bone injury is another issue that is starting to arise. Inadequate renal patients have a disease called renal osteodystrophy, caused by an increase in PTH and a decrease in vitamin D production, a hormone that controls the amount of calcium in the bones and blood. The result is the demineralization of the bones, which are beginning to get weak and sick.

Stage III is the stage in which patients must start treatment and be accompanied by a nephrologist, since from this point on there is usually a relatively rapid progression of renal failure if there is no adequate treatment.

Stage 4

Patients with creatinine clearance between 15 and 29 ml/min.

This is the stage for pre-dialysis. This is when the first symptoms start to appear, and several changes are shown in laboratory tests.

The patient has high phosphorus and PTH levels, established anaemia, low blood pH (increased blood acidity), high potassium levels, weight loss and signs of malnutrition, worsening hypertension, weakened bone levels, increased risk of heart disease, decreased libido, decreased appetite, fatigue, etc.

The patient may not notice weight loss due to fluid retention, as the weight may remain the same or even increase. The patient loses fat and muscle mass but retains fluids, and small edema in the legs may develop.

The patient should already be ready for hemodialysis at this stage, indicating the construction of an arteriovenous fistula.

Stage 5

Patients with a creatinine clearance of less than 15 ml/min.

This is referred to as an end-stage renal failure. The kidney no longer performs basic functions below 15–10 ml/min, and the commencement of dialysis is indicated. At this point that patients, called uremia symptoms, begin to experience symptoms of kidney failure.

If dialysis is not started, the condition progresses. Those who do not die from cardiac arrhythmias may progress with pulmonary edema or mental changes, such as disorientation, seizure crisis, and even coma. Although they are still able to urinate, the volume is not so large, and the patient begins to develop large edema. Blood pressure is out of control, and blood potassium levels are so high that they can cause cardiac arrhythmias and death. The patient has already lost a lot of weight and cannot eat well. You experience nausea and vomiting, especially in the morning. You get tired easily and anaemia, if not already being treated, is usually at dangerous levels.

When ultrasound of the kidneys is performed, they are usually already atrophied, with reduced sizes.

Some patients manage to reach stage V with a few signs and symptoms. Despite little symptomatology, they show numerous laboratory alterations. The longer the start of dialysis is delayed; the worse will be the bone, cardiac lesions, malnutrition, and the risk of malignant arrhythmias. Often, the first and only symptom of end-stage renal failure is sudden death.

Kidney Diseases—Causes, Symptoms, Diagnosis, and Treatment

Kidney disease is a collection of various diseases that attack this organ. Their common denominator is a serious threat to health and life and difficulty in diagnosis in the first phase. What else is worth knowing about them?

Kidney Disease—Causes

It is difficult to identify only one cause of kidney disease because it depends on the patient we are dealing with. However, it cannot be denied that one of the most serious negligence is the patient. Some illnesses result from untreated infections, bacteria cause others, and others are the result of a lack of concern for the kidneys in everyday life. Of course, the causes of kidney disease are not always known to us. Sometimes we can only guess at them, and sometimes they are caused by an inappropriate response from the immune system, and doctors have no idea how to change the way it works. It also happens that problems with the kidneys are a consequence of improper intimate hygiene, which women should be especially aware of.

Kidney Disease—Threat

Care for the urinary tract should be something obvious to us, regardless of our age and gender, but some groups of people are at greater risk of developing it than others. Reference is made to the particular risk in the context of older people who, due to their age, already have a reduced efficiency characteristic of the immune system. The risk is particularly high in the context of men, especially if they have a problem with prostate enlargement; however, women and people with hypertension are also at risk, regardless of their age. It is also worth monitoring the kidneys' condition, knowing that medications are often taken, especially antibiotics and painkillers.

Kidney Disease—Symptoms

Asking about the symptoms of kidney disease is one of the things that makes doctors embarrassed. This is not only because each disease has a slightly different course, but also because it is characterized by development without any symptoms alarming the patient. Worse still, even when health problems do arise, you cannot be sure that they will be properly diagnosed. The signals sent by the body can be so non-specific that patients are treated for months for a different disease than the one they are struggling with.

However, we were to indicate those signals, the appearance of which should raise our alertness, we should first pay attention to changes in the urine. We usually see those that affect its smell, but changes can also affect its appearance, colour, and transparency.

Other symptoms depend primarily on the disease we are dealing with. It sometimes happens that the only alarm signal is increased blood pressure, malaise, drowsiness, and headaches. Even symptoms as surprising as peeling of the skin and vomiting can show kidney problems, and sometimes the patient smells the ammonia, not in the urine but the mouth.

Kidney Disease—Diagnosis

Kidney diseases can be difficult to diagnose, so it's no wonder that prevention is of great importance in treating them. Untreated, they can hinder our normal functioning, sometimes making it impossible. Therefore, it is not worth risking the disease, especially since its diagnosis at an early stage does not have to be difficult. This goal can be achieved with a general urine test. Your GP should issue a referral for them, but you should not give up the examination, even if you do not have time to go for the appropriate document. Urine can be tested in almost any analytical laboratory, and because the testing is not complicated, it is also inexpensive.

Usually, the analysis of protein in the urine is analyzed. Still, it is also important for the doctor to determine whether and in what quantity there are white and red blood cells. It is also good to observe the state of the urine yourself so that the power to intervene immediately, as soon as we notice the first disturbing changes.

Kidney Disease—Treatment

The treatment of kidney diseases depends primarily on the disease we are dealing with in a given case. The doctor also considers the general condition of the patient, which is of great importance in the case of older people. Pharmacological treatment is usually of key importance, as it allows to eliminate the symptoms and causes of the disease. However, the patient is also expected to change the diet, give up stimulants, and take greater care of the quantity and quality of fluids consumed.

Unfortunately, while pharmacology is increasingly effective, it is also failing under certain circumstances. In the case of uremia, we are dealing with long-term treatment, which often ends with dialysis, and a patient with kidney cancer must take into account that at some point, removing an infected organ will be the only chance for him to protect himself from death. Many patients benefit from pyelonephritis by having an operation during which a catheter is inserted into the bladder. Systematic medical control is also recommended in each case.

Kidney Disease—Consequences of Neglect

Not all patients decide to treat kidney diseases, even if they are chronic. Therefore, it is worth remembering that the consequence of this approach is usually a renal failure. When it occurs, more and more poisonous substances appear in the patient's body when the blood is not cleaned properly, causing problems with the proper functioning of other organs, including such important ones as the heart, liver, brain, and endocrine glands. In extreme cases, the patient's carelessness leads to the need for dialysis and even a kidney transplant.

Chapter Three:
Benefits of Following a Renal Diet

You need a meal plan that includes a kidney diet if you have a kidney disorder. You will help stay healthy if you notice what you eat and drink. The facts in this section apply to individuals with kidney disease who are not treated with dialysis.

We are all different, and our nutritional needs are different for everyone. Talk to your kidney dietician (a diet and nutrition expert for kidney disease patients) to see which meal scheme works best for you.

Ask your doctor to help find a nutritionist. Private insurance and Medicare policies can help pay for dietary appointments.

As part of the hygienic-dietary measures, nutritional advice should be the first recommendation to the patient. Dietary care has always been considered important in chronic kidney disease (CKD), both as a renoprotective antiproteinuric measure in the predialysis stage, as to prevent overweight and malnutrition in all stages, especially the latter in dialysis patients. The first premise is to guarantee adequate caloric, protein, and mineral support. Never the price to pay for a supposedly adequate diet must be insufficient nutrition. The nutrient recommendations should be adapted to the ideal weight—not real—and corrected for energy expenditure and physical activity of the patient.

Why Is It So Important to Follow a Meal Plan?

The things we were eating and drinking can affect your health. Maintaining a healthy weight and eating a balanced diet low in salt and fat can help control blood pressure. People with diabetes can help control blood sugar levels by choosing very carefully what to eat and drink. Controlling blood pressure and diabetes can help prevent kidney disease from getting worse.

A kidney diet helps prevent damage to the kidneys. The kidney diet limits certain foods and prevents the minerals of those foods from accumulating in the body.

Fundamentals of the Renal Diet

With all meal plans, including the renal diet, it is necessary to track the number of specific nutrients you consume, such as:

- Calories
- Protein
- Grease
- Carbohydrates
- Etc.

To make sure you're getting the right amount of these nutrients, you need to eat and drink the correct portion sizes. All the information you need to track your consumption is a "nutritional information" label.

Use the nutrition information section on meal labels to learn more about the foods you eat. The nutrition information will tell you how much protein, carbohydrates, fat, and sodium are in each serving of that meal. This can help you choose foods rich in the nutrients you need and low in the nutrients you should limit.

When you look at nutrition data, some key areas will give you the information you need:

Calorie

The calories you eat and drink are the source of your body's energy. Protein, carbohydrates, and dietary fats are the products of calories. The calorie required depends on your age, sex, body size, and level of activity.

You can adjust your calorie consumption by weight. Some people restrict their calories; others must eat more calories.

Protein

Protein is one of the body's fundamental components. To grow, heal, and remain healthy, the body needs protein. Skin, hair, and nails could be weakened by too little protein. But there is too much protein. To improve your health and mood, the amount of protein you eat may have to be adjusted.

The number of protein you should consume depends on your body size, level of activity, and health problems. Some doctors recommend people with kidney disease to limit their protein or change their protein source. This is because a high-protein diet can hinder kidney function and cause damage.

Protein intake recommendations vary depending on the stage of the patient. In ACKD, a moderate restriction of protein intake is recommended; in dialysis patients, intakes should be higher to compensate for the catabolic nature of the technique.

Find out which foods are low and high in protein. Remember that just because a meal is low in protein does not mean that you can consume it in high amounts.

Low protein meals	High protein meals
Bread	Red meat
Fruits	Chicken
Vegetables	Fish
Pasta and rice	Eggs

Protein Restriction in ACKD

The kidney is the natural route of elimination of nitrogenous products. It is based on the fact that unlike sugars and fats whose final product is H_2O and CO_2, the final product of protein metabolism is nitrogen, which is eliminated mainly by the kidneys in the form of urea. With renal failure progression, these nitrogenous products (together with phosphates, sulphates, and organic acids) accumulate in proportion to the loss of renal function. This not only gave rise to the principle of protein restriction but also to the urea kinetic model to establish the dialysis dose. Protein restriction has been prevalent for decades (since 1918) and has been the cornerstone of treatment when dialysis did not exist.

Hydration

Hydration in ACKD is discussed in an extensive format elsewhere. For dialysis patients, it is recommended to drink as much liquid as is eliminated with the urine in this period, plus an additional 500–750cc. Regarding the patient's weight, the interdialytic gain should not exceed 4–5% of their dry weight. In PD, the fluid balance is continuous, but the peritoneal ultrafiltration capacity is limited, so a moderate fluid restriction and adjusted to the peritoneal balances are recommended.

Salt Intake

The limitation of saline intake is a classic indication, both in patients with ACKD and renal replacement therapy. It is important to prevent hydro saline retention, an adjunct in controlling blood pressure, and even reduces proteinuria and facilitates the effect of renin-angiotensin axis blockers.

We must consider it very important to be able to verify the saline intake objectively to favour the adherence of this prescription. The most affordable method of monitoring saline intake is urinary sodium excretion, and we must emphasize the importance of measuring urinary sodium during routine office visits. Now, is urinary sodium useful as an indicator of salt intake? The answer is not easy to find in the literature, and the information must be sought in the classical books of human physiology. Under normal conditions, faecal sodium excretion is less than 0.5% of the intestinal content of the ion, thanks to its rapid and effective absorption by the intestinal mucosa. Therefore, if we consider that the intestine absorbs almost all of the sodium ingested; urinary sodium elimination is a good reflection of salt intake. Although there is always the risk of inadequate 24-hour urine collection, several studies have highlighted that it is the most practical method to verify salt intake.

Grease

To stay healthy, you need some fat in your food plan. Fat gives you energy and helps you eat certain vitamins. However, too much fat can lead to heart and weight gain. Try to limit your dietary fat and, if possible, select healthier fats.

The healthiest fat or "good" fat is called unsaturated fat. Examples of unsaturated fats include:

- Olive oil
- Peanut oil
- Corn oil

Unsaturated fat can contribute to lower cholesterol levels. Try to eat unsaturated fats if you need to gain weight. Limit unsaturated fats in your food plan if you need to lose weight. Modesty is the key, as always. There may be too many problems with 'good' fat.

Saturated fat, also called "bad" fat, may increase your heart disease risk and cholesterol level. Saturated fat examples contain:

- Butter
- Lard
- Shortening
- Meats

Limit these fats in your eating plan. Choose healthy, unsaturated fats instead. Cutting the amount of fat in meats and removing the skin from chicken or turkey can also limit saturated fat.

Trans fats should also be avoided. This kind of fat increases your 'bad' cholesterol and decreases your 'good' cholesterol. If this occurs, your heart disease may be more likely to lead to kidney damage.

Sodium

Sodium (salt) is a mineral found in almost every food. Too much sodium can thirst, which can cause bloating and increase blood pressure. This can damage your kidneys and make it harder for your heart to work.

One of the best ways to stay healthy is to limit your sodium intake. To control the sodium in your meal plan:

- Do not add salt to your food when you are cooking or eating. Try to cook with fresh herbs, lemon juice, or unsalted spices.
- Choose fresh or frozen vegetables from canned vegetables. If you are using canned vegetables, drain and rinse to remove the salt before cooking or eating.
- Avoid processed meats like ham, bacon, hot dogs or chorizo, and lunch meats.
- Eat fresh fruits and vegetables instead of cookies or other salty snacks.
- Avoid canned soups and frozen meals that are high in sodium.
- Avoid foods such as olives and pickles that have been pickled.
- Limit high-sodium condiments such as soya sauce, barbecue sauce, or ketchup.

Important! Important! Be careful with salt substitutes or "lower sodium" foods. A lot of salt substitutes are high in potassium. Too much potassium can be hazardous if you have kidney disease. Work with your dietitian to find foods that are low in sodium and potassium.

Portions

It is a great beginning to choose healthy foods, but eating too much can be an issue. The other component of a healthy diet is the control of portions or watching how much you eat.

To control portions:

- On all foods, check the label for nutrition facts and learn the serving size. Most bundles have more than one serving. A 20-ounce bottle of soda, for example, is two and a half servings. With nutrition facts labels, fresh foods, like fruits and vegetables, do not come. Ask your dietician for a list of fresh foods for nutrition and advice on measuring portions correctly.

- Eat slowly and when you are not hungry anymore, stop eating. It takes your stomach approximately 20 minutes to tell your brain that it is already full. You may eat more than you need if you eat too quickly.

- When doing something else, such as watching TV or driving, avoid eating. You do not know how much you have eaten when you are distracted.

- Do not eat from the food package directly. Take a portion of food out, instead, and put the bag or box at a distance.

Controlling portion sizes is important to any meal plan. It is even more important on a kidney diet because you may need to limit how much you eat or drink.

What Is the Difference Between Kidney Diets?

Waste and fluids build up in your body when your kidneys are not working as well as they should. This additional fluid and waste can cause heart, bone, and other health problems over time. A kidney diet meal plan can restrict the number of certain minerals and fluids you consume. This can avoid building up and causing problems with waste and extra fluids.

Depending on your stage of kidney disease, it will depend on how strict you must be with your plan. There may be little or no limit to what you eat or drink in the early stages of kidney disease. As time goes by and your kidney disease gets worse, your doctor may recommend limiting:

- Potassium
- The match

- Liquids

Potassium

Potassium is a mineral that is present in nearly all foods. For your muscles to work, your body needs some level of potassium, but too much potassium can be hazardous. Your potassium level can be very high or very low when your kidneys are not working well. Muscle cramps, problems with how your heartbeats, and muscle weakness can be caused by having too much or not enough potassium.

You can restrict how much potassium you eat if you have kidney disease. Ask your doctor or nutritionist if you should limit your consumption of potassium.

Find out which foods contain high and low potassium levels. Your nutritionist can help you understand how healthy it is to eat small amounts of your favourite high-potassium foods.

Eat this (Low potassium foods)	Instead of (Foods high in potassium)
Apples, grapes, strawberries, pineapple, and ploughing,	Avocados (avocado), bananas, melons, oranges, plums. and raisins.
Cauliflower, onions, bell peppers, radishes, summer squash, and lettuce	Artichokes, pumpkin, bananas, spinach, potatoes. and tomatoes.
Pita, tortillas, and white bread,	Bran and granola products.
Beef, chicken, and white rice,	Beans, brown or wild rice (baked, black, pinto, etc.)

Match

Phosphorus has been found in nearly all foods as a mineral. Works to maintain your bones healthy, using calcium and vitamin D. Healthy kidneys keep phosphorus in the body at the right level. Phosphorus can build up if your kidneys do not work well. In your blood, too much phosphorus can easily cause bones to break.

There must be phosphorus limits for many people with renal diseases. Please ask your doctor if phosphorus should be restricted.

Your doctor may prescribe a medicine called a phosphorus binder, depending on your stage of kidney disease. This can prevent your blood from developing phosphorus. You may have to look at the amount of phosphorus that you are eating in your diet.

To get an idea of how to make healthy choices if you need to limit phosphorus in your diet, use the table below

Eat this (Low phosphorus meals)	Instead of this (Foods high in phosphorus)
Italian, French, or sourdough bread.	Whole grain bread.
Corn or rice cereals and cream of wheat.	Bran and oat cereals.
Unsalted popcorn.	Dried fruits and sunflower seeds.
Light-colour soda or lemonade.	Dark colour sodas.

Our bodies need survival water, but you may not need water so much if you have kidney disease. This is why they do not remove extra fluids as they should if their kidneys are damaged. Too many fluids can be dangerous in your body. High blood pressure, heart failure, and swelling can occur. The additional fluids that you collect near your lungs can make breathing difficult.

Your doctor may request that you limit the number of fluids you drink, depending on the kidney disease stage and your treatment. You will need to limit how much you take if your doctor asks you to do this. Some foods containing water will also have to be cut off. Soups and foods melting have plenty of water, like icing cream and gelatine. In water, too, a lot of fruit and vegetables are high.

To control how much you drink, you have to limit fluids, measure the quantities of liquid and drink from small glasses. To prevent thirst, limit the amount of salt. You may feel thirsty sometimes. You can do the following to help alleviate thirst:

- Chew gum.

- Rinse your mouth.

- Suck on an ice cube, mint or hard caramel (remember to choose a sugar-free caramel if you have diabetes).

Special Dietary Concerns

Vitamins

Following a diet plan with a kidney diet may prevent your body from getting enough vitamins and minerals you need. To help you get the right levels of vitamins and minerals, your dietician may suggest a supplement created for people with kidney disease.

Therapists or dieticians may also suggest a special type of vitamin D, folic acid, or iron pill to help prevent some side effects typical of kidney disease, such as bone disease and anaemia.

Regular use of many vitamins may not be healthy for you if you have kidney disease. They may contain much or too little vitamin.

After Diabetic Kidney Meal

Should you have diabetes, you need to control blood sugar levels to prevent damage to the kidneys. A doctor or nutritionist can help you create a meal plan that enables you to control blood sugar levels while limiting sodium, phosphorus, potassium, and water.

Diabetes educators can also learn to control blood sugar levels. Ask your doctor to introduce you to a diabetes educator in your area. Private insurance and Medicare can help you pay for reservations with diabetic educators.

Chapter Four:
How to Improve Kidney Function

One of the most important organs in your body is your kidneys. In regulating your blood, blood volume, blood pressure, and blood pH, they have important functions. In the form of urine, they are also responsible for filtering blood and the excretion of waste. To enhance your overall health, and reduce your chances of getting sick, take great care of your kidneys. Many things can go wrong, but you may be less likely to suffer from things like kidney stones, kidney infections, or failure if you follow a few simple tips.

Eat Healthily

Eat a Balanced Diet

This is one of the main factors in good overall health, and your kidneys are no exception. Avoid fatty and salty foods. Consume lots of fresh fruits and vegetables. If you're not sure how to put together a balanced diet, you can use the food pyramid, which divides foods into different groups.

Public health experts criticized the original food pyramid, and you can now find the newer, revised version. Here, healthy foods are combined with other aspects, such as weight control.

Lower the Amount of Salt in Your Diet

It is very normal for people to consume too much salt or sodium in their diet. Foods high in salt or sodium can be particularly bad for the kidneys. High levels of sodium can lead to high blood pressure. Over time, high blood pressure can damage your kidneys and make you more susceptible to serious kidney disease.

- Choose fresh rather than pre-packaged foods. As a result, you'll typically consume less sodium.

- If you buy pre-packaged foods, make sure that the packaging says 'no extra salt' or something similar.
- Get in the habit of studying food labels and finding out the sodium content of each food.

Eat "Kidney-Friendly" Foods

Adhering to a balanced and healthy diet should be a priority, but some foods are particularly beneficial for your kidney function. Foods with antioxidants—usually fruits and vegetables—can help boost the overall health of your kidneys. Some of the best vegetables to have on your shopping list are cabbage and cauliflower, berries (especially cranberries), red peppers, and onions.

- Although cranberries are very good food for you, store-bought cranberry juice can be high in sugar.
- Asparagus is especially good for your kidneys.

Drink Healthily

Drink a Lot of Water

Staying hydrated has a beneficial effect on your health. If you are well hydrated, your urine is more diluted and thus supports healthy kidney function. Some doctors recommend eight glasses of water a day, but in some cases, more than this amount is recommended. Water supports the flushing of toxins from the body. Moisturizing the body well with fluid, makes this task for the kidneys and helps regulate body temperature better.

Drink Water Regularly

Drink water frequently throughout the day, and don't just swallow half a litre at a time, twice a day. The kidneys regulate the fluid in your body. They can do their job more easily if you drink small amounts frequently.

Only Drink Alcohol in Moderation

Consuming large amounts of alcohol may have serious negative consequences for the functioning of your kidneys. Filtering harmful substances out of your blood is one of the primary jobs of the kidneys. Alcohol is one of the most dangerous compounds that your kidneys have to deal with. The functioning of your kidneys can be negatively affected by excessive alcohol consumption.

Alcohol dries you out, and that can also harm your kidneys, whereas good hydration positively affects kidney function.

Weight Control and Regular Exercise

Control Your Weight

It is important to maintain a healthy weight. Being overweight can increase your blood pressure, which can put even more strain on your kidneys. Stick to a good diet and exercise regularly to maintain a healthy weight and keep your blood pressure low.

Obesity can also lead to diabetes. Diabetes with high blood pressure is the two main causes of kidney disease.

Train Enough

Active life and exercise have several positive consequences for your health and play an important role in weight management. Exercise is also helpful for blood circulation and mobility. The kidneys are relieved in their task of regulating the blood in the body. Exercising regularly can also help prevent diabetes and stabilize your blood pressure. This will reduce the stress on your kidneys and lower the risk of kidney disease.

- Suppose you are not used to exercising regularly. In that case, it is important to incorporate these activities into your daily routine so that you can soon see the long-term benefits and improvements in kidney function. Achieving this can be difficult if you are a very busy person or a rather easy-going person, but you should make an effort to find the right path.

- Find a sport or activity that you enjoy. This is probably the best way for someone to enjoy exercise if they're not used to it.

- Training together with friends or your partner can be much funnier and more relaxing if you don't want to join a club or team.

Get a Good Supply of Vitamin D When You Exercise Outdoors

Kidney disease can be related to a vitamin D deficit. Activating vitamin D is one of the kidneys' jobs. By getting vitamin D from the sun, you can reduce the pressure on your kidneys.

- To promote kidney function, you need to be in the sun for at least 15 minutes a day.

- Vitamin D also regulates calcium and phosphorus levels in the body.

The Emergence of Kidney Disease

Understand How the Kidneys Work

You can first read a little and educate yourself. Learn how the kidneys operate and what their functions are. In keeping your blood healthy, the kidneys play a major role and thus enable important nutrient transport in the body. They also protect you against disease and balance the pH. If you think about it, you will realise how important your overall health is to the health and good functioning of the kidneys.

Know-How Kidney Disease Occurs

After you understand the function and importance of healthy kidneys, you can learn a little more about how kidney disease is caused. The two most common triggers are diabetes and high blood pressure. There are numerous other causes, including poisoning or injury and trauma. Kidney disease, for example, can develop after a particularly severe blow to the kidneys.

Some pain relievers can cause kidney problems with long-term, regular use. If you are taking these drugs, you should check with your doctor.

Ask Your Parents if There Have Been Other Cases of Kidney Disease in the Family

Kidney disease is often hereditary. If your family is prone to kidney disease, you may be at slightly higher risk. If so, you can seek advice from your doctor so that you can avoid inheritable kidney disease as much as possible.

How to Avoid Dialysis

- Optimized blood pressure always setting below 140/90 mmHg; after consultation with the attending physician, possibly even below. This usually does not work without taking medication.

- **Sufficient fluid intake:** approx. 2 to 2.5 litres per day. Every liquid is included, including coffee, tea and soups.

- **Pay attention to your diet:** a high protein intake puts a strain on the kidneys. Therefore, the diet should be "normalized" for protein, with 0.8 grams of protein per kilogram of body weight and day (approx. 64 grams for 80 kilograms of body weight).

- **Also important:** save table salt, no more than five to six grams a day

- Moderate physical activity with light endurance training, 30 to 60 minutes five times a week.

- **No smoking:** Smoking damages the kidneys!

- If you have diabetes, ensure that your blood sugar is controlled well. Values that are too high damage to the kidney.

- Avoid certain pain medications, such as ibuprofen and diclofenac. If in doubt, ask the kidney specialist (nephrologist).

- As little contrast media (containing iodine) as possible should be used during X-ray examinations.

- Regular checks by the nephrologist.

Steps to Control Chronic Kidney Failure

Seek Treatment for Hypertension

The pressure is now considered the leading cause of chronic renal failure. According to nephrologist Nestor Scho, professor at Unifesp, the increase in blood pressure damages the blood vessels of the kidneys and may cause hypertensive nephropathy. "This way, the organ becomes overloaded, and little by little loses its filtering capacity," he explains. Taking care of hypertension is essential even when it is not the cause of chronic renal failure, as it becomes even more important in the advanced stage of the disease.

Control of Diabetes

"Diabetes is the second leading cause of chronic renal failure," says nephrologist Lucio Roberto Requião Moura of Hospital Israelita Albert Einstein. This is because the disease triggers the so-called diabetic nephropathy, a change in kidney vessels that leads to a protein loss in the urine. Also, diabetes favours atherosclerosis, the formation of plaque fat in the arteries that hinders the filtration work of the kidneys. Over time, more and more toxic substances are trapped in the body, leading to death. Therefore, one way to detect the problem is to do urine tests to find out if the protein is being eliminated. Those already diagnosed with diabetes need to be more aware of their kidney health.

Watch the Weight

Overweight people (discover your ideal weight) have a higher risk of developing hypertension and diabetes, which is reason enough not to let the scale hand rise, says nephrologist Lucio. Added to this is that obesity alters the way blood reaches the kidneys by the influence of certain hormones, overloading the organ. More so, being overweight is a risk factor for high cholesterol and triglycerides.

Adapt Your Diet

When it comes to food, analysing the underlying disease that triggered kidney failure is critical. If it is diabetes, for example, the diet should be the right diet for those with diabetes. If it is hypertension, then there should be reduced salt intake. "However, in general, it is recommended that the patient avoid excessive protein intake, especially of animal origin, which gives rise to toxic elements in the body that would make the kidneys work harder," explains nephrologist Nestor. In specific cases of insufficiency yet, there may be retention of potassium in the body. Patients with this problem need to prepare food in a way that causes them to release some of this nutrient. Vegetables, for example, need to be cooked.

Inquire About Medications

Self-medication is dangerous even for healthy people. For those with kidney failure, however, use without proper medical evaluation can accelerate kidney deterioration. "The most dangerous are non-hormonal anti-inflammatory drugs," warns nephrologist Lucio. Therefore, explain your problem at the beginning of every medical appointment to avoid aggravating the disease.

Way to Drink Alcohol

Although no studies prove the isolated relationship between alcohol intake and chronic renal failure, alcohol abuse compromises the functioning of the body as a whole. Thus, it is recommended to handle your consumption. However, if you are going to have a drink nephrologist Nestor advises to opt for wine. "It contains antioxidants that can help eliminate concentrated toxins in the body," he says

Put Out the Cigarette

"Cigarettes are responsible for worsening blood pressure levels and are still involved with hormonal changes that worsen kidney function," explains nephrologist Lucio. Also, smoking triggers a vasoconstriction effect, decreasing the volume of blood filtered by the kidneys. In this case, there is no moderation option. The patient must end the addiction.

Practice Exercises

The last recommended care for chronic kidney failure sufferers is regular exercise. "It prevents diabetes, hypertension, obesity, among other problems, and improves circulation and kidney function," says nephrologist Nestor. According to him, any activity is already better than physical inactivity. Still, it is always recommended to seek training that pleases the patient not to feel discouraged over time.

Chapter Five:
Foods to Avoid if You Have Bad Kidney

The kidneys are the small, bean-like organs responsible for performing some of the most important bodily functions. For example, the kidneys are responsible for generating important hormones, eliminating waste when urinating, filtering the blood, and maintaining a balance of fluids and minerals.

Kidney disease or damage renders the kidneys unfit to perform any of these functions, wreaking havoc on the human body. Several risk factors increase the likelihood of kidney disease, for example, excessive hypertension and uncontrolled diabetes. Some other common causes of kidney disease include heart disease, HIV infection, alcoholism, and hepatitis C.

Once the kidneys become damaged and lose their ability to fulfil their responsibility, an excessive accumulation of fluids, minerals, and waste products begins to accumulate within the bloodstream. However, you can prevent further damage and increase your kidney's ability to function by eating an effective diet that contains foods that do not harm the kidneys and help reduce the accumulation of waste, minerals, and fluids.

Dietary recommendations and restrictions generally depend on the stage of kidney disease or the extent of damage that has occurred and vary according to it. Compared to patients in the late stage of kidney damage or kidney failure, patients who experience the early symptoms of chronic kidney disease will receive markedly different dietary restrictions and recommendations.

Patients who experience late-stage kidney failure symptoms, and are treated with dialysis, a treatment that removes fluid build-up and removes waste products, will receive different dietary recommendations. Most patients suffering from symptoms of late-stage or end-stage renal failure have no choice but to adopt a diet suitable for the kidneys and avoid foods that threaten to create an excessive accumulation of harmful chemicals or nutrients in the bloodstream.

Among patients with chronic kidney disease, the kidneys cannot adequately remove excess phosphorus, potassium, and sodium from the bloodstream. Therefore, these minerals put them at risk for elevated blood levels. An effective kidney diet revolves around consuming foods and beverages that will ensure that your sodium and potassium intake does not exceed 2000 mg per day, while phosphorus intake cannot increase more than 1000 mg per day.

Kidneys that are damaged tend to have a hard time filtering waste products that are made when protein is metabolized. Therefore, patients with stage 1–4 symptoms of chronic kidney disease should reduce their protein intake. However, patients taking dialysis treatment with end-stage renal failure require increased protein intake.

Foods that you must eliminate for an effective kidney diet:

Cola Soda

Calories and sugar are loaded with sugar-filled sodas and artificially flavoured colas, and they also contain a variety of phosphorus-brimming harmful additives, especially dark coloured drinks.

Phosphorus is used by most food manufacturers to process food and beverage products, specifically to enhance their taste, increase shelf life, and reduce discolouration. Research shows that artificially added phosphorus, compared to phosphorus consumed by animal meat, plants, or other natural sources, tends to be much more absorbable by the body.

Artificial phosphorus additives tend to have a composition different from natural phosphorus and are therefore not protein-bound. As a type of salt that is easily absorbed from the intestinal tract, these additives are present. In the ingredient list for products, artificially added phosphorous is included, but regulations do not require food manufacturers to specify the exact amount of additive phosphorous added to their product.

The additive phosphor present is highly dependent on the variety you are consuming, but research reveals that most dark coloured glues contain around 50–100mg of additive phosphorus. Therefore, they must be strictly eliminated from an effective kidney diet.

Avocados

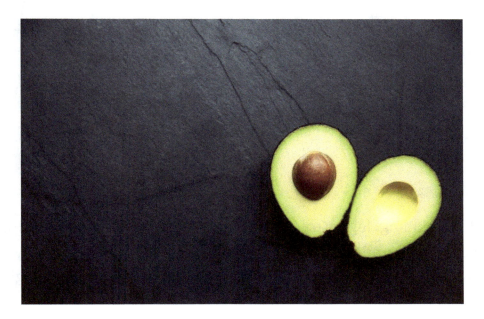

Avocados are nutritional superfoods that are considered immensely beneficial and essential due to these rich concentrations of heart-healing antioxidants, fats, and fibre. However, despite being such a healthy staple, they are a dangerous food for people struggling with kidney disease.

This is mainly due to the incredibly rich potassium concentration found in avocados. For example, a 150-grams serving of avocados contains an alarmingly high amount of 727mg of potassium, which is twice the potassium amount present in a medium-sized banana.

Think about it; one cup of avocado can provide you with more than 37% of your daily potassium restriction of 2000mg. Therefore, it is highly recommended to eliminate avocados and avocado-based products, such as guacamole.

Canned Food

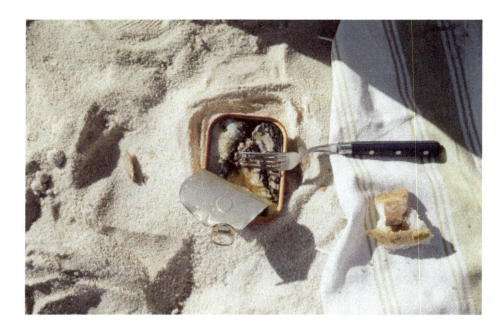

Canned foods, including legumes, fruits, vegetables, sauces, and soups, are often brought home due to undeniable convenience and affordability. Many people who commonly buy these canned foods are unfamiliar with the alarmingly high amounts of sodium in these foods.

High amounts of salt are added to varieties of canned food as a preservative to improve flavour and increase the shelf life of the product. Due to the excessively high density of sodium present in most canned foods, it is highly recommended that patients with kidney damage avoid them altogether or limit their portion sizes if they add them to their diets.

It is always a healthier option to choose varieties of canned foods that are low in sodium or labelled "no added salt." You can also reduce sodium density by 30–80% simply by rinsing and draining canned foods. This technique works best with canned legumes and tuna.

Wholemeal Bread

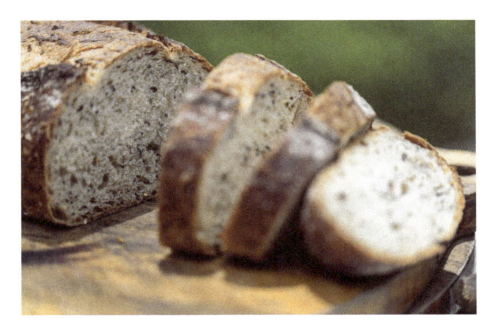

Whole wheat bread is widely considered the healthiest option for a perfectly balanced diet, and more refined and processed white flour bread is discouraged due to its lack of essential nutrients. However, when you have kidney disease or damage, it can be difficult to choose the right variety of bread that doesn't aggravate your symptoms.

Even whole wheat bread is a much more nutritious option due to its rich fiber concentration, but kidney-impaired patients are strongly advised to choose white bread over whole grain varieties. You see, whole wheat bread contains a high concentration of potassium and phosphorus, and the higher the concentration of bran and whole grains, the higher the concentration of these two nutrients.

For example, a 30-gram serving of whole wheat bread will provide you with 69mg of potassium and about 57mg of phosphorus. On the other hand, a one-ounce serving of white bread will only provide you with 28mg of potassium and phosphorus. Just keep in mind that most processed bread and packaged bread products, whether whole wheat or white, also contain large amounts of sodium.

It is strongly recommended to select the pieces of bread after comparing and examining the nutrition labels of various varieties. Make sure to choose a variety that is low in sodium, and it's also important to cut down on your portions and limit your intake as much as you can.

Integral Rice

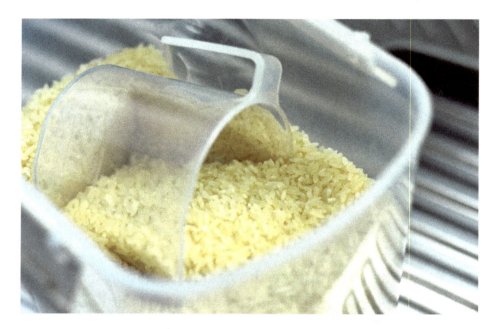

Like whole wheat bread and other products, brown rice is also a whole grain and therefore contains a much higher density of potassium and phosphorus than white rice. For example, a cup of cooked brown rice will provide you with 154mg of potassium and 150mg of phosphorus. On the other hand, a cup of cooked rice will only provide you with 54mg of potassium and 69mg of phosphorus.

You can add brown rice to your diet as long as you can control your portion sizes and eat them occasionally by balancing it with other foods that are low in phosphorus and potassium. It is highly recommended to choose grains that are low in phosphorus, such as buckwheat, couscous and pearl barley, which are much safer alternatives for an effective kidney diet.

Bananas

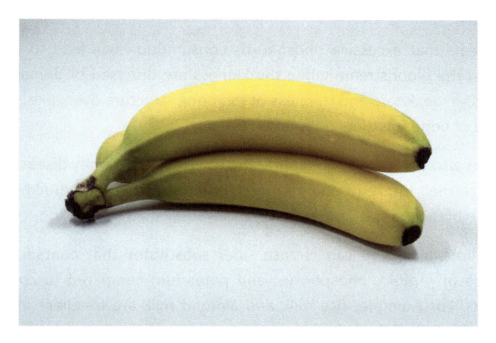

Bananas are popular for packing an incredibly rich concentration of potassium. Although they naturally contain lower sodium concentrations, a medium-sized banana will give you 422mg of potassium. If you are in the habit of consuming more than two bananas a day, it can be extremely difficult to keep your daily potassium intake below 2000mg.

If you like to eat tropical fruits, be aware that almost all varieties contain extremely rich potassium concentrations. However, pineapples have a considerably lower potassium density compared to other tropical fruits.

Dairy Products

Dairy products contain a rich concentration of nutrients and vitamins; they are an essential part of a healthy and balanced diet. But dairy products are also rich in potassium, phosphorus, and protein, making them a hazardous dietary ingredient for kidney disease patients.

In patients with kidney disease, regular consumption of various dairy products and other foods rich in phosphorus can be hazardous to bone health. This is a surprise because the calcium content is widely recommended for strengthening the muscles and bone structure in dairy products, particularly milk.

Research reveals that excessive phosphorus consumption will lead to a build-up of phosphorus in the bloodstream when the kidneys are diseased or damaged. This will lead to excessive weakness and thinness of the bone structure over time, leading to an increased risk of bone fractures or breaks.

Dairy products also tend to be high in protein. Patients with kidney disease should take steps to reduce their intake of dairy products to prevent excessive build-up of protein residues in the bloodstream.

Instead of whole milk, you can choose safer substitutes that contain much lower concentrations of protein, phosphorus, and potassium compared to cow's milk and dairy products. For example, rice milk and almond milk are excellent alternatives to whole milk in the diet of the kidneys.

Oranges and Orange Juice

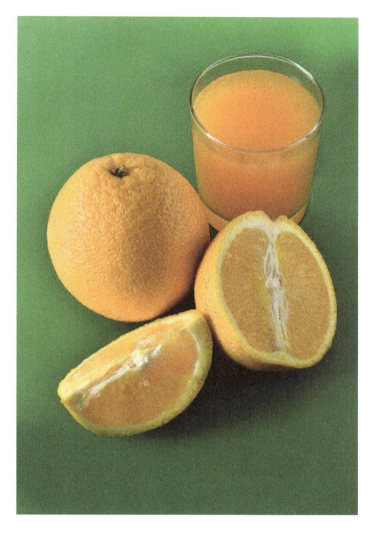

Even though oranges and freshly squeezed orange juice are among the richest and healthiest sources of vitamin C, these citrusy delicacies also contain an incredibly high concentration of potassium. A large orange can provide you with an alarming 333mg of potassium. But orange juice contains a higher density.

Considering their dangerously high potassium concentration, it is best to avoid oranges and orange juice, and if you must add it to your kidney diet, reduce the portions. Instead of oranges, you can select healthier fruits that contain lower potassium densities, such as grapes, blueberries, and apples.

Processed Meats

A large body of research establishes a direct association between the regular consumption of processed meats and risk factors for chronic diseases. Processed meats are considered one of the least healthy staples because they accumulate an alarmingly high preserves concentration.

Processed meats are canned, dried, salted, or cured meats, for example, sausage, bacon, pepperoni, jerky, etc. Processed meats are packed with dangerously high amounts of salt, which enhance flavour and preserve the flavour for longer shelf life. Additionally, these processed meats also contain a high density of protein. If your doctor has specifically instructed you to reduce your protein intake, consuming processed meats regularly is an unhealthy habit for you.

Pickles, Olives, and Sauce

Pickles, seasonings, and processed olives are the most commonly consumed types of cured or pickled foods. The pickling and curing process involves the addition of unusually large and unhealthy amounts of salts.

Processed olives that are fermented and cured to make their tasteless bitter are also dipped in salt to alter the bitter taste. Five green pickled olives contain an alarming 195mg of sodium, which turns out to be a dangerous serving of sodium in such a small serving. Most supermarkets and grocery stores offer low-sodium varieties of olives, seasonings, and pickles that tend to pack less salt than their traditional counterparts. However, keep in mind that even low sodium varieties tend to accumulate large amounts of sodium.

Therefore, it is best to restrict your consumption of processed olives, pickles, and condiments, and if you have to consume them, consume very small amounts.

Apricots

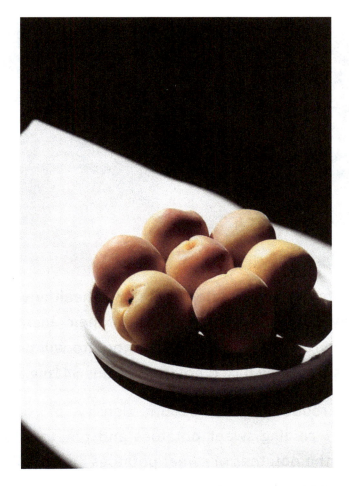

Apricots are a powerful superfood as they pack an incredibly rich concentration of various essential nutrients and minerals; including fibre, vitamin A, and vitamin C. Unfortunately for patients with kidney damage; they also contain dangerously high amounts of potassium. Just one cup of raw apricots contains a whopping 427mg of potassium.

When apricots are dried, their potassium content becomes more concentrated and strengthened. A one-cup serving of dried apricots contains more than 1,500mg of potassium.

It is important to eliminate apricots, particularly dried apricots, to enjoy effective results from a successful kidney diet.

Potatoes and Sweet Potatoes

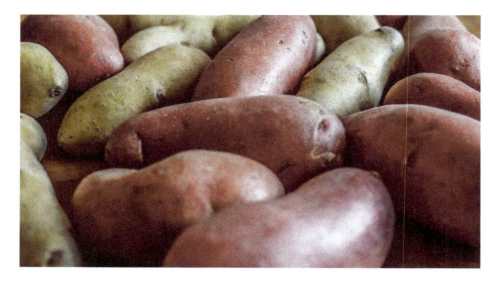

Even though sweet potatoes and potatoes are not unhealthy vegetables, they can be harmful to a kidney-damaged patient due to their incredibly rich potassium concentration. Consuming a medium-sized baked potato will provide you with 610mg of potassium, while a small-sized baked potato contains 541mg of potassium.

Fortunately, we can reduce the potassium density of several potassium-filled vegetables and fruits, including sweet potatoes and potatoes, simply by soaking or leaching them. Cutting the potatoes or sweet potatoes into small pieces like cubes and boiling them for at least 10–15 minutes will reduce the potassium concentration by 50%.

Another impressive method to reduce potassium content is to put potatoes in a large pot of water for more than four hours before baking or cooking. It causes a noticeable reduction in potassium content compared to potatoes that are not soaked before cooking. This technique is known as potassium leaching and is more popularly known as the double cooking method.

Just be sure to note that while the potassium leaching method helps reduce the potassium content in potatoes, this technique does not remove the potassium completely. Even twice-cooked potatoes and boiled sweet potatoes pack up significant amounts of potassium content. Therefore, it is highly recommended to consume moderately conscious portions so that your potassium levels remain under control.

Tomatoes

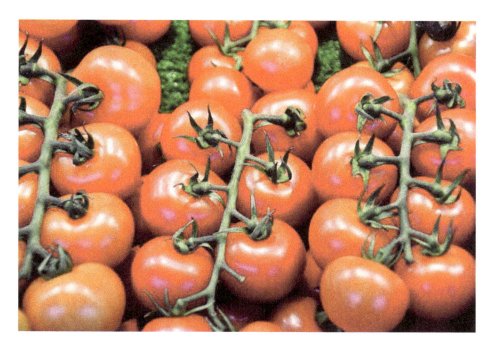

Despite containing a beneficial concentration of several essential nutrients, tomatoes are another vegetable loaded with a dangerously high concentration of potassium, so they are not a favourite ingredient for an effective kidney diet. Tomatoes are commonly added to sauces and meals and are also served raw in salads or sandwiches and stewed in soups.

Be careful about consuming tomatoes, as just one cup of tomato sauce can contain more than 900mg of potassium.

You can easily alternate tomatoes with roasted red bell peppers to create a flavorful red sauce that will provide you with various nutrients and a considerably lower potassium density.

Packaged, Instant, and Prepared Meals

Processed, ready-to-eat foods and all packaged varieties are major sources of excessive amounts of sodium in our daily diet. These prepared and packaged meals contain excessive salt amounts with no trace nutrients and are best eliminated from a kidney diet.

Most varieties of packaged and ready-made meals typically contain highly processed ingredients and are therefore full of sodium. Some popular consumer varieties include microwaveable meals, frozen pizzas, and packets of instant noodles. In addition to being high in sodium, these processed foods are loaded with unhealthy fats and lack essential body needs.

Swiss Chard, Spinach, and Beet Greens

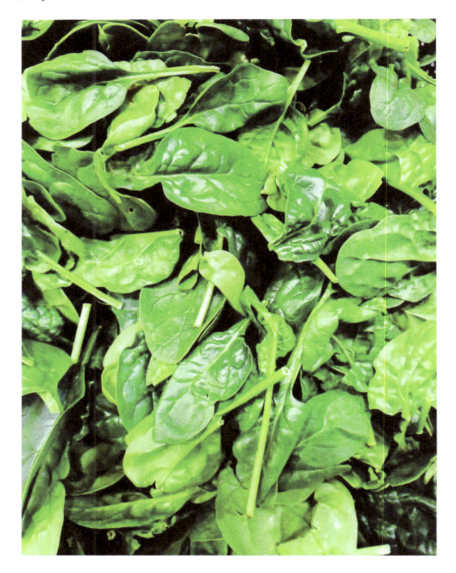

One of the healthiest green leafy vegetables, containing incredibly high concentrations of nutrients and minerals, particularly potassium, is spinach, beet greens, and Swiss chard. They deliver a potassium concentration that ranges from 140–290mg in a one-cup serving when consumed raw. However, their potassium content increases when these leafy vegetables are cooked, even though their size is reduced.

As long as you're eating moderately portion-conscious, it's okay to add raw spinach, green beets, and Swiss chard to your salads, and avoid cooked meals of these leafy greens altogether to avoid a potassium overdose.

Dates, Raisins, and Plums

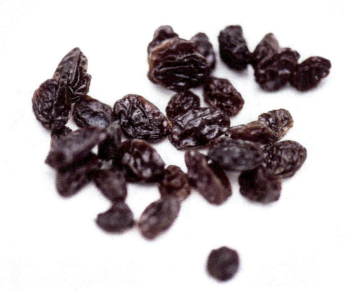

Prunes, raisins, and dates are the most widely consumed dried fruits and are popularly added to many packaged baked goods and desserts. Research reveals that when fruits are allowed to dry, all of their nutrients, including their potassium concentration, are converted to a concentrated form.

For example, a one-cup serving of plums contains 1,274mg of potassium, approximately five times the potassium concentration supplied by a cup of raw plums. Even worse is the potassium density of dates, which accumulate a whopping 668mg of potassium with just four dates.

Increasing your potassium intake is dangerous for patients suffering from kidney damage. It is highly recommended to eliminate or at least reduce your potassium intake to enjoy effective results from your kidney diet. Plums, dates, and raisins simply cannot be included on the list due to their dangerously high potassium concentration.

Pretzels, Chips, and Cookies

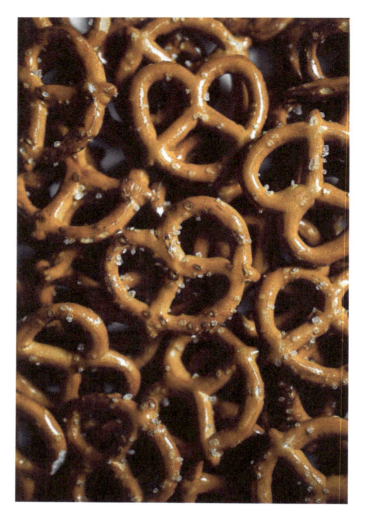

Crackers, potato chips, and pretzels are very low in nutrients and contain dangerously unhealthy salt amounts. Besides, it is very easy to consume large amounts of these foods, causing you to consume much more salt than you intend to consume.

Patients with kidney disease should reduce their intake of phosphorus, potassium, and sodium, as their reduction is strongly related to the reduction and management of symptoms.

Due to the absence of goodies on the menu, it can be extremely difficult to go on a kidney diet, making eating very restrictive and disappointing. However, foods that contain dangerously high amounts of phosphorus, sodium, and potassium should be avoided.

For assistance in designing a diet plan specific to your kidney condition, be sure to consult your renal specialist, nutritionist, or dietitian. The dietary restrictions and suggestions you should follow will naturally depend on the severity of your symptoms and the extent to which your body has suffered kidney damage.

Best Foods for People with Kidney Disease

Restrictions in diet depend a lot on the degree of kidney damage. Generally, to protect these organs, we ask to limit the consumption of sodium, the main component of salt, potassium and phosphorus. Proteins should also be wary of, as their waste products can strain the kidneys. Here are the best foods for people with kidney disease.

1. **Cauliflowers:** Cauliflower has many benefits. They contain fibre, vitamins C, K, and the B group. They are also anti-inflammatory and can be used in place of potatoes.

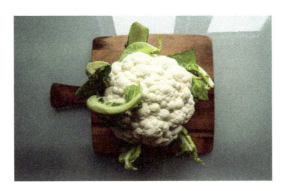

One cup of cooked cauliflower contains:

- **Sodium:** 19mg
- **Potassium:** 176mg
- **Phosphorus:** 40mg

2. **Blueberries:** Blueberries are a treasure trove of well-being. In particular, they contain antioxidants, such as anthocyanins, which protect us from cardiovascular disease, certain types of cancer, cognitive decline, and diabetes.

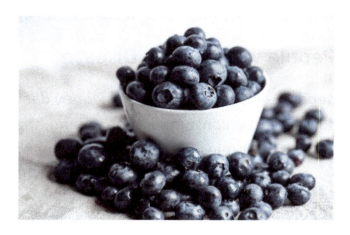

One cup of blueberries contains:

- **Sodium:** 1.5mg
- **Potassium:** 114mg
- **Phosphorus:** 18mg

3. **Sea bass:** Bass contains high-quality protein and valuable Omega 3s, which help reduce inflammation and can help counter the risk of cognitive decline, depression, and anxiety. Unlike many other fish that are rich in phosphorus, sea bass has little of it.

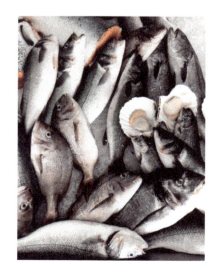

One hundred grams of cooked sea bass contain:

- **Sodium:** 80mg
- **Potassium:** 290mg
- **Phosphorus:** 230mg

4. **Black grapes:** Grapes are full of vitamin C and antioxidants capable of reducing inflammation. Furthermore, the berries are particularly rich in resveratrol, a precious flavonoid that helps the heart and brain.

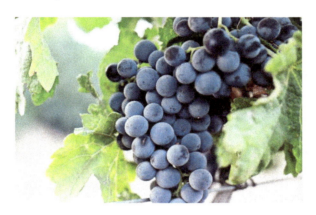

Half a cup of black grapes contains:

- **Sodium:** 1.5mg
- **Potassium:** 144mg
- **Phosphorus:** 15mg

5. **Egg whites:** Although egg yolks are very nutritious, they contain high amounts of phosphorus, which is not beneficial to those with delicate kidneys. Egg whites, on the other hand, are an excellent choice.

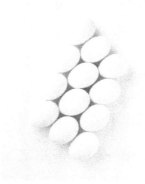

Two egg whites contain:

- **Sodium:** 110mg
- **Potassium:** 108mg
- **Phosphorus:** 10mg

Garlic: They can be a tasty alternative to the use of salt. They also contain a good dose of manganese, vitamins C and B6, and contain molecules with anti-inflammatory properties.

Three cloves of garlic contain:

- **Sodium:** 1.5mg
- **Potassium:** 36mg
- **Phosphorus:** 14mg

6. **Buckwheat:** Grains very often contain a lot of phosphorus, but buckwheat is an exception. It contains B vitamins, magnesium, iron, and fibre. Since it does not contain gluten, it is also ideal for those who have celiac disease.

Half a cup of buckwheat contains:

- **Sodium:** 3.5mg
- **Potassium:** 74mg

- **Phosphorus:** 59mg

7. **Extra virgin olive oil:** It is healthy and phosphorus-free.

30 grams of olive oil contain:

- **Sodium:** 0.6mg
- **Potassium:** 0.3mg
- **Phosphorus:** 0mg

8. **Broken wheat:** Known as bulgur, cracked wheat is an ancient kidney-friendly grain. It is a good strong in B vitamins, magnesium, iron, and manganese. It also contains fibre and protein.

One hundred grams of bulgur contains:

- **Sodium:** 4.5mg
- **Potassium:** 62mg
- **Phosphorus:** 36mg

9. **Cabbage:** The cabbage belongs to a cruciferous cauliflower-like tree. It is rich in antioxidants, minerals, and vitamins.

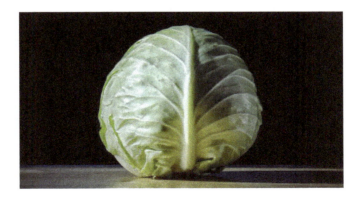

One cup of cooked cabbage contains:

- **Sodium:** 13mg
- **Potassium:** 119mg

- **Phosphorus:** 18mg

10. **Skinless chicken:** Chicken is kidney-friendly if cooked and then eaten skinless. We never try to buy cooked chicken because it is enriched with sodium and phosphorus.

One hundred grams of skinless chicken contains:

- **Sodium:** 70mg
- **Potassium:** 230mg
- **Phosphorus:** 200mg

11. **Peppers:** Peppers contain an impressive amount of nutrients and little potassium, unlike many vegetables. They are rich in vitamin C; they also contain vitamin A.

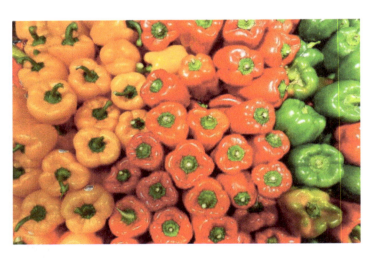

A small pepper contains:

- **Sodium:** 3mg
- **Potassium:** 156mg
- **Phosphorus:** 19mg

12. Onions: They are also an excellent trick to give flavour to foods using a little salt and, therefore, sodium. Besides, onions are rich in vitamins C and B, manganese, and fibre.

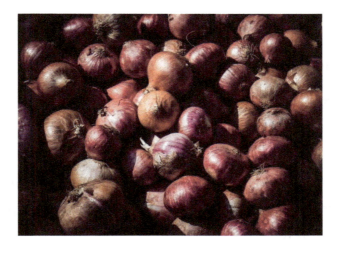

A small onion contains:

- **Sodium:** 3mg
- **Potassium:** 102mg
- **Phosphorus:** 20mg

13. Rocket salad: It is a salad with a lot of flavours and many benefits. It is rich in vitamin K, manganese, and calcium.

It also contains nitrates, which help lower blood pressure.

One cup of rocket contains:

- **Sodium:** 6mg
- **Potassium:** 74mg
- **Phosphorus:** 10mg

14. **Macadamia nuts:** Nuts are high in phosphorus. Macadamia nuts are not, as well as being rich in healthy fats, B vitamins, magnesium, copper, iron, and manganese.

30 grams of macadamia nuts contain:

- **Sodium:** 1.4mg
- **Potassium:** 103mg
- **Phosphorus:** 53mg

15. **Radishes:** They have little potassium and phosphorus, unlike vegetables in general. They are also rich in vitamin C and antioxidants. Their spicy flavour helps to use even less salt.

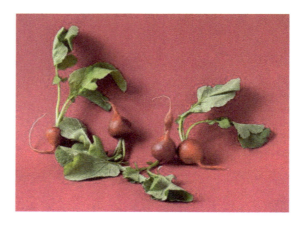

Half a cup of radishes contains:

- **Sodium:** 23mg
- **Potassium:** 135mg
- **Phosphorus:** 12mg

16. **Turnips:** It has vitamins C, B6, manganese, and calcium; they are perfect allies for the kidneys.

Half a cup of cooked turnips contains:

- **Sodium:** 12.5mg
- **Potassium:** 138mg
- **Phosphorus:** 20mg

17. **Pineapple:** It usually contains a lot of potassium. Pineapple does not. It is also rich in fibre, B vitamins, manganese and bromelain, which reduces inflammation.

One cup of pineapple chunks contains

- **Sodium:** 2mg
- **Potassium:** 180mg
- **Phosphorus:** 13mg

18. **Redberry:** Cranberries are especially valuable for the urinary tract and kidneys. They contain phytonutrients that make sure that bacteria do not remain in the urinary tract.

One hundred grams of cranberries contain:

- **Sodium:** 2mg
- **Potassium:** 85mg
- **Phosphorus:** 13mg

19. **Shiitake mushrooms:** They are a very tasty ingredient, rich in B vitamins, copper, manganese, and selenium.

One cup of cooked Shiitake contains:

- **Sodium:** 6mg
- **Potassium:** 170mg
- **Phosphorus:** 42mg

Daily Tips to Boost Your Kidney Function

The diet for kidney dialysis helps maintain the balance of electrolytes, minerals, and fluids in dialysis patients. The special diet is important because all waste products are not effectively removed by dialysis alone. Between dialysis treatments, these waste products can also build up.

Most patients with dialysis urinate very little or not, and fluid restriction between treatments is very important. Without urination, fluid in the heart, lungs, and ankles will build up in the body and cause excess fluid.

Dialysis seeks to eliminate the waste of excess water and nitrogen, thereby reducing renal failure symptoms. Dialysis can be used temporarily as a permanent, life-sustaining treatment if the client has acute renal failure or if the client has chronic renal failure. In the latter case, dialysis must continue for the remainder of the patient's life unless successful kidney transplantation is performed.

The kidney dialysis diet is also used in combination with dialysis to control uremia and physically prepare the client to receive a transplanted kidney. Usually, dialysis is necessary until a suitable kidney donor kidney is found to keep the client alive. If the transplanted kidney does not immediately function properly, dialysis may help prevent uremia until the kidney starts functioning properly.

Here are some general guidelines on what to do before or after the commencement of dialysis treatment:

- Eat meals periodically.
- In your diet, include plenty of variety. This will provide you with essential nutrients, such as protein, calories, vitamins, and minerals. They keep you well-nourished with these nutrients.
- Eat some high-fibre foods, such as cereals and whole grain bread.
- Just eat a moderate amount of fat.
- If you have high blood pressure, avoid adding extra salt to your food.

Chapter Six:
Diet for Chronic Kidney Disease

Removing waste and purifying the blood is the major role of the kidneys. In addition to this, in removing excess water, minerals, and chemicals, the kidney plays an important role. Therefore, it regulates the balance throughout the body of water and mineral salts such as sodium, potassium, calcium, phosphorus, and bicarbonates.

The regulation of water and electrolytes may be disturbed in patients with chronic kidney disease (CKD). This is why the hydro-electrolytic balance can be seriously disrupted by the usual intake of liquids, salt, and potassium. Patients suffering from CKD should adjust their diet according to the doctor and dietitian's recommendations to reduce the work of the kidneys already suffering and avoid disturbances in the fluid and electrolyte balance. For MRCs, there is no fixed regime. Each patient has a diet adapted to his or her clinical condition, the stage of his or her renal failure, and the presence or lack of other health problems. Dietary advice for the same patient should be reviewed and regularly reviewed.

The objectives of diet in case of CKD are:

- Slow chronic renal disease progression, thereby delaying dialysis requirements.
- Reduce the toxicity of excess urea in the blood.
- Maintain optimal nutritional status and prevent weight loss.
- Reduce the risk of fluid and electrolyte imbalance.
- Reduce the risk of cardiovascular disease.

High-Calorie Intake

The details of calorie intake in patients with CKD are as follows:

High-Calorie Intake

For daily activities, the body needs calories to maintain a steady temperature, to grow taller, and to have a healthy body weight. Fat and carbohydrates primarily provide calories. In a CKD patient, the daily calorie requirement is between 35 and 40 kcal/kg of body weight per day. Proteins will be used to compensate for the caloric needs if this caloric intake is not properly ensured. This breakdown of proteins can have adverse effects on the body, such as malnutrition and increased toxic waste production. In patients with CKD, therefore, it is essential to provide an adequate amount of calories. The patient's calorie needs must be calculated according to his ideal weight and not according to his actual weight. The weight, particularly in patients with malnutrition or diabetes, may be lower or higher than the ideal weight.

Carbohydrate

The body's primary source of calories is carbohydrates. They are found in sugar, honey, cakes, candies and drinks, wheat, rice, grains, potatoes, fruits, and vegetables.

Diabetics and obese individuals need to decrease their intake of carbohydrates. In grains such as whole wheat, whole rice, and Indian millets such as finger millet (nachni, ragi) sorghum, bajra, or pearl millet, which also contain fibres, it is best to use complex or slow carbohydrates. A large proportion of carbohydrates, associated with a small amount of simple or fast carbohydrates such as sugar and should not exceed 20 per cent of the total intake of carbohydrates, should constitute complex carbohydrates.

Lipids

Fat provides twice as much energy as carbohydrates or protein and is an important source of calories for the body. Lipids or unsaturated fatty acids (good lipids) are better than lipids or saturated fatty acids contained in red meat, whole milk, butter, cheese, bacon, poultry, Indian clarified butter or ghee, and coconuts, such as olive oil, peanut oil, rapeseed oil, safflower oil, sunflower oil, fish and nuts. Your saturated fat and cholesterol intake needs to be reduced because they can lead to heart disease and kidney damage.

The proportions of monounsaturated lipids and polyunsaturated lipids should be paid attention to among unsaturated lipids. It is harmful to have an excessive intake of omega-6 polyunsaturated fatty acids and a high Omega-6/Omega-3 ratio, while the body benefits from a low Omega-6/Omega-3 ratio. Better than pure oil, blends of vegetable oils achieve the goal. Doughnut-based foods, crisps, Vanaspati/Dalda Ghee (palm oil vegetable butter), marketed pastries are potentially harmful and should be avoided.

Protein Restriction

Protein is essential for repairing and maintaining tissue in the body. They also help in the healing of wounds and the fight against infections.

Protein restriction reduces the rate of deterioration of kidney function, thus delaying the need for dialysis and kidney transplantation. But excessive protein restrictions should be avoided. Lack of appetite is common with CKD. The combination of protein restriction and lack of appetite can quickly lead to nutritional deficiency, weight loss, lack of strength, and high susceptibility to infections, leading to death. In India, most Indians are vegetarians. Even non-vegetarians don't take animal products every day. The amount of protein is closely linked at the socio-economic level. It remains far from the recommendations of the Indian Council of Medical Research, which recommends 1 gram per kilo of weight per day. Consequently, the protein restriction of 0.8g/kg per day recommended in MRCs to slow its progression is limited. More emphasis should be placed on the quality of the proteins to consume. Attention should be paid to the complex proteins (0.4–0.6g/kg) contained in curdled milk, paneer cheese, soy milk powder, dry soybean pieces and soybeans, white cheese, egg, etc., and for non-vegetarians, egg white or fatty fish of which we can take small qualities.

Water intake

Why Should Patients with CKD Take Precautions Regarding Water Intake?

By removing the excess water in the form of urine, the kidneys play a major role in keeping the body's water supply constant. In CKD patients, urine volume decreases as kidney function deteriorates.

With the appearance of puffiness of the face, edema of the legs and hands, arterial hypertension, the decrease in the volume of urine causes retention and suddenly an excess of fluid in the body. Dyspnea is due to the accumulation of fluids in the lungs. It may kill the patient if these symptoms are not taken care of.

What Are the Signs of Excess Fluids?

Excess water is still called hyperhydration. The most common signs are oedema, ascites (accumulation of fluid in the abdomen), dyspnea, and severe weight gain over a short period.

What Precautions Should Patients with CKD Take to Control Fluid Intake?

To avoid excess or lack of water, take as many fluids as advised by the attending physician. The volume of fluid intake varies from patient to patient and should be calculated based on the urine volume and hydration status of each patient with CKD.

How Many Fluids Are Allowed in Patients with Chronic Kidney Disease?

- In patients without edema and with the correct urine volume, no restriction is advised. But in patients with chronic kidney disease, taking plenty of water to protect the kidneys is a misconception.

- Patients with edema and decreased urinary volume are required to reduce fluid intake. To reduce edema, the number of fluids allowed should be less than the 24-hour urine volume.

- To avoid excess or lack of water, it is advisable to drink the amount of urine increased by 500ml. The 500ml that we add roughly covers the water losses through sweat and breathing.

Why Do Patients with CKD Need to Weigh and Record Themselves Daily?

It is to monitor the state of hydration and early detect an imbalance. Bodyweight remains constant when water intake is made as recommended. Sudden weight gain indicates water overload linked to intake greater than necessary. Weight gain warns patients to reduce their fluid intake. Weight loss usually occurs after diuretic treatment and reduced fluid intake.

Helpful Tips to Reduce Water Intake

Reducing water intake is hard, but these tips can help you do it.

- Weigh yourself at the set time of the day and readjust your water intake according to your weight.

- The doctor will inform you of the number of fluids to take daily. Therefore, we calculate and measure the amount of water drunk every day. Remember that the water intake does not only concern water but also tea, coffee, milk, curds, butter, juices, ice cream, cold drinks, soups including thin dal, etc. When calculating the volume of water drunk, you will have to take into account the water intake in your diet. Be wary of watermelons, grapes, lettuce, tomatoes, celery, sauces, gelatins, frozen foods such as ice cream, etc., because they are rich in water.

- Cut back on salt, spices, and fried foods in your diet because they increase the feeling of thirst, causing you to consume more fluids.

- Drink only when you are thirsty. Don't be in the habit of drinking or accompanying someone who drinks.

- If you are thirsty, take a small amount of water or try ice cream. Take an ice cube and suck it. Ice stays longer in the mouth than liquids and therefore gives more satisfaction than the same water volume. Remember to count ice cubes as drunk water. To make the calculations easier, you will freeze the required quantity in the ice cube trays.

- To keep the mouth hydrated, you can gargle with water but without swallowing it. Dry mouth can also be combated by chewing gum, sucking on hard candy, lemon wedges, or mint, or using liquid toothpaste to moisturize the mouth.

- Always use a small glass for drinking; this will help you limit your water intake.

- Take your medicine after meals with the water you drink at these times; this will save you additional water to swallow your tablets.

- The patient must attend to work. An unoccupied person often feels the need to drink water.

- Hyperglycemia in diabetics increases the feeling of thirst. It is, therefore, essential to have strict glycemic control.

- During the hot season, thirst increases. It is therefore recommended to live in the comfort of freshness to avoid the thirst.

How do you measure and consume precisely the prescribed daily amount of fluids?

- The exact amount of water prescribed by the attending physician per day should be placed in a container.

- The patient should remember that he or she is not allowed to drink more than the container's contents over and over again throughout the day.

- Each time the patient drinks something else, he must assess the amount and deduct it from the water in his container.

- Once the container has been emptied, the patient should know that he will not drink anything more during the current day. Therefore, it is advisable to distribute the authorized quantity of water throughout the day to avoid adding more.

- This control method should be done every day.

- Thanks to this simple but effective method, the authorized quantity of water per day is respected.

Salt Restriction (Sodium)

Why Do Patients with CKD Need to Take Less Salt?

Dietary Sodium is important for maintaining blood volume and blood pressure. The kidneys play an important role in regulating sodium. In patients with CKD, the kidneys cannot remove excess sodium and water.

Thus, sodium and water are found in excess in these patients. Excess sodium increases thirst, edema, dyspnea, and high blood pressure. To prevent or reduce these problems, patients with CKD should reduce their salt intake.

What Is the Difference Between Salt and Sodium?

The words salt and sodium are often used synonymously. The salt that everyone knows is sodium chloride, which contains 40% sodium. Salt is the main source but not the only source of sodium in our diet.

There are a few other sources of sodium in our diet like:

- **Sodium Alginate:** Used in ice creams and milk chocolates.
- **Sodium Bicarbonate:** Used as baking powder and sodas.
- **Sodium Benzoate:** Used as a preservative in sauces.
- **Sodium Citrate:** Used to enhance the taste of gelatin, desserts, and beverages.
- **Sodium Nitrate:** Used in preserving and as a colouring agent in certain dishes.
- **Sodium Saccharide:** Used as a sweetener.
- **Sodium Sulphite:** Used to prevent discolouration of dried fruits.

The compounds mentioned above contain sodium without having a salty taste. The sodium is "hidden" in it.

How Much Salt Should We Take?

The amount of salt ingested by Indians on average is 6 to 8g/day. Patients with CKD should take the amount recommended by their doctor. Patients with CKD with edema and high blood pressure are often required to take around 3g/day.

What Foods Are High in Sodium?

Foods high in sodium are:

- Table salt (salt that everyone knows), yeast.

- Papadum, salted pickles, salted chutney sauces, sauces, mixes for seasoning or chaat masala and sambharas.

- Bakery products like cookies, cakes, pizzas, and bread.

- Foods containing yeast such as certain Indian foods such as ganthiyas, pakoras or vegetable fritters, dhoklas made from fermented rice paste, handvo or Gujarat cake, samosa fritters, ragda patties, dahi vadas, etc.

- Wafers, crisps, popcorn, savory donuts, salted dried fruits such as pistachios, peanuts, canned foods, etc.

- Butter and salted cheeses.

- Instant foods like noodles, spaghetti, macaroni, cornflakes, etc.

- Vegetables such as cabbage, cauliflower, fenugreek, beets, radish, coriander leaves, etc.

- Drinks such as salted lassi, masala soda, lemon lemonade, and coconut water.

- Medicines such as sodium bicarbonate, antacids, and laxatives.

- Foods for non-vegetarians like meat, chicken, animal offal like kidneys, liver, and brains.

- Seafood such as crabs, lobsters, oysters, shrimp and fatty fish such as columbi, kurang, crab, mackerel, and dried fish.

Practical Advice to Reduce Your Salt Intake

- Reduce salt intake and avoid adding salt to dishes made with yeast. Prepare your meals without salt and just add the authorized amount. This is the best way to control the amount of salt ingested per day.

- Do not serve savoury dishes or savoury seasonings at the table, and do not leave table salt on the dining table. Do not add salt to your salads, rice, curds, Indian bread like chapatti, parathas and bhakri, etc.

- Carefully read the contents of dishes sold in stores. Look not just for salt, but for anything that may contain sodium. Read the instructions carefully and look instead for sodium-free or "sodium-free" or low-salt "low sodium" products.

- Beware of the sodium contained in drugs.

- Boil foods high in sodium and discard the cooking water. This can reduce the sodium content.

- To make the diet tasty little salted, we can add garlic, onion, lemon juice, amchur, bay leaves, tamarind paste, vinegar, cinnamon, cardamom, cloves, saffron, green peppers, nutmeg, black pepper, cumin, fennel, poppy seeds, etc.

- Warning! Avoid salt substitutes because they can contain a lot of potassium. This potassium from salt substitutes may elevate the blood potassium level in patients with CKD and be dangerous.

- Do not drink the softened water. In the process of making this water, calcium is replaced by sodium. Water purified by reverse osmosis is less rich in mineral salts, including sodium.

- If you are at a restaurant, choose foods where there is less sodium.

Potassium Restriction

Why Are Patients with CKD Advised to Eat a Low Potassium Diet?

Potassium is important for the body. The body needs it for the proper functioning of muscles and nerves and regularly beating the heart.

Normally, the potassium level is kept constant through a balance between food intake and the elimination of excess by the kidney. This elimination can be disturbed in the event of CKD, which can lead to an increase in the level of potassium in the body (hyperkalemia) between two dialysis sessions. The risk of hyperkalemia is lower with peritoneal dialysis compared to hemodialysis. The risk is different in the two groups because the dialysis is continuous in peritoneal dialysis while it is intermittent in the case of hemodialysis.

Hyperkalemia can cause muscle fatigue and irregular heartbeat, which can be dangerous. If the hyperkalemia is very severe, the heart may stop beating suddenly and cause sudden death. Hyperkalemia can be life threatening without prior manifestations (the silent killer).

To avoid these serious consequences of hyperkalemia, patients with CKD are forced to reduce their potassium intake.

What Is the Normal Level of Potassium in the Blood? At What Rate Is It Considered High?

- The level of potassium in the blood is 3.5 mEq/l to 5.0mEq/l.
- When the potassium level is between 5.0 to 6.0 mEq/l, it requires a diet modification.
- When the potassium level exceeds 6.0 mEq/l, it becomes dangerous and requires intervention to lower it.
- When the potassium level is above 7.0 mEq/l, it can be life-threatening and requires urgent treatment.

Classification of Foods According to Their Potassium Content

To maintain the correct level of potassium in the blood, certain foods should be avoided as prescribed by the doctor. Based on the potassium content of these foods, they are classified into three categories (very high, high and low in potassium).

- **Very high in potassium:** more than 200mg/100g of food.
- **Rich in potassium:** 100 to 200mg/100g of food.
- **Low in potassium:** less than 100mg/100g of food.

Foods very high in potassium:

- **Fruits:** Fresh apricots, amla, bananas, coconut, custard, guava, pomegranate, currant, kiwi, mango, melon, oranges, papaya, peaches, apples, plums, and sapoti.
- **Vegetables:** Amaranth, eggplant, broccoli, pumpkin, cyamopsis, colocasia, coriander, mushrooms, spinach, beans, yams, raw papaya, drumstick, potatoes, tomatoes, and sweet potatoes.
- **Dried fruits:** Almonds, dates, hazelnuts, dried figs, raisins, and walnuts.
- **Cereals:** Wheat, Bajra, or ragi flour.
- **Dried vegetables:** Beans and dried lentils of different colours.
- **Mixed spices:** Cumin seeds, coriander seeds, dried red chilli, and fenugreek seeds.
- **Non-Vegetable Foods:** Fish such as anchovies, mackerel, crabs, and beef, shellfish such as shrimp, lobster.
- **Drinks:** Bournvita, beer, buffalo milk, coconut water, condensed milk, drinking chocolate, fresh fruit juice, soft drinks, rasam soup, soup, cow's milk, and wine.
- **Miscellaneous:** Chocolate, cadbury, chocolate cake, chocolate ice cream, Lona salt (substitute salt), crisps, and tomato sauce.

Foods high in Potassium:

- **Fruits:** Ripe cherries, lime, lychee, watermelon, pear, and grapes.
- **Vegetables:** Bananas, beets, carrots, safflower leaves, bitter gourd, cabbage, celery, cauliflower, okra, green beans, raw mango, onions, radishes, green peas, and sweet corn.
- **Cereals:** Barley, all-purpose flour (maida), millet jowar, wheat-based noodles, and vermicelli, rice flakes (pressed rice, poha).
- **Non-vegetarian dishes:** Cital, hilsa (fish), katla, magur, liver.
- **Drinks:** White cheese.

Foods low in potassium:

- **Fruits:** Pineapple, cherries, lemon, strawberries, raspberries, and apples (rose apple).
- **Vegetables:** Garlic, pumpkin, squash, broad beans, calabash (turiya), cucumber, fenugreek leaves (methi), lettuce, and sweet pepper.
- **Cereals:** Rice, rava, and wheat semolina.
- **Legumes:** Green peas.
- **Non-vegetarian dishes:** Beef, lamb, pork, chicken, and eggs.
- **Drinks:** Coffee, coca-cola, Fanta, lemonade, lemon juice, Limca, Rimzim, and sodas.
- **Miscellaneous:** Cloves, dry ginger, honey, mint leaves, mustard, nutmeg, black pepper, and vinegar.

Practical Tips for Reducing Potassium in the Diet

- Take one fruit per day, preferably low in potassium.
- Take a cup of tea or coffee a day.

- Vegetables rich in potassium should only be taken after reducing potassium (as explained below).

- Avoid coconut water, fruit juices, and foods rich in potassium (list above).

- Among the foods that contain potassium, choose those that contain the least potassium when possible.

- Potassium restriction is necessary not only in patients with CKD on predialysis but also after the initiation of dialysis.

How Do You Reduce the Potassium in Vegetables?

- Peel and cut the vegetable foods into small pieces, wash them with lukewarm running water, and put them in a large bowl.

- Fill the bowl with hot water (4 to 5 times the food volume) and let it soak for at least an hour.

- After soaking the food for 2–3 hours, rinse it 3 times with lukewarm water.

- Boil the vegetables with plenty of water that you throw in at the end.

- Foods thus boiled can be prepared as desired.

- Thus, you can reduce the potassium level in some foods, but not completely. Therefore, it is preferable to avoid foods rich in potassium or to take it in small quantities.

- As these foods lose vitamins during cooking, vitamin supplements will be taken as prescribed.

Special tips for reducing potassium in potatoes:

- Cut the potato into small pieces, thus maximizing the surface of the vegetable in contact with the water.

- It is the temperature of the water used to soak or boil the potatoes that make the difference.

- Using plenty of water for soaking or boiling is beneficial.

The Restrictive Phosphorus Diet

Why Should Patients with CKD Eat a Low Phosphorus Diet?

- Phosphorus is an essential mineral for strong bones in the body. Often, the excess phosphorus supplied by the diet is eliminated in the urine, thus maintaining a balanced phosphorus level.

- Normal blood phosphorus values range from 4.0 to 5.5mg/dl.

- In patients with CKD, excess phosphorus from the diet is not excreted in the urine, and the phosphorus level increases in the blood. The increase in phosphorus in the blood causes a release of calcium from the bones, thus causing their fragility.

- The increase in phosphorus in the blood causes other manifestations such as itching, the fatigue of muscles and bones, bone pain, joint pain. Stiff bones increase the risk of fractures.

What Foods Are Rich in Phosphorus That Should Be Avoided or Reduced?

Foods very rich in phosphorus are:

- **Milk and derived products:** butter, cheese, chocolate, condensed milk, ice cream, milkshake or milkshake, cheese, or paneer.

- **Dried fruits:** cashew nuts, almonds, pistachios, dry coconut, walnut.

- **Cold drinks:** Coke, Fanta, Mazza, Frooti, beer.

- Carrots, colocasia leaves, corn, peanuts, fresh peas, sweet potato

- **Animal proteins:** meat, chicken, fish, and eggs.

High Intake of Vitamins and Fibres

Patients with CKD suffer from inadequate vitamin intake during pre-dialysis due to severe diet, the way food is prepared to get rid of excess potassium, and lack of appetite. Besides, some vitamins, especially those soluble in water such as vitamins B, C and folic acid, etc., are lost during dialysis.

To compensate for inadequate intake and increased losses, patients with renal failure often require supplementation with water-soluble vitamins and trace elements. A diet rich in fibre is beneficial in CKD patients. Thus, it is recommended that these patients take a lot of fresh vegetables and fruits, which are rich in fibres and vitamins.

Designing a Daily Diet

For MRC patients, the daily ration of food and liquids is planned by the dietitian in collaboration and according to the advice of nephrologists.

The main principles of the ration concern:

- **Fluid intake (including liquid from food):** water restriction should be done according to the doctor's advice. The weight curve should be plotted daily.
- **Carbohydrates:** to ensure an adequate caloric intake with cereals, the patient can take the sugar or glucose in food, provided he does not have diabetes.
- **Protein:** Milk, grains, meats, and eggs are the main source of protein. CKD patients who are not on dialysis should reduce the protein intake in their ration. It is recommended to take 0.8 grams per pound of body weight per day. Once dialysis is started, patients need more protein (especially those on peritoneal dialysis). One should avoid eating proteins of animal origin such as meat, chicken, and fish, foods that are also rich in potassium and phosphorus. All proteins of animal origin can be harmful to CKD patients.
- **Lipids:** the rate of lipids (fat) in food intake must be reduced, but the total elimination of butter, clarified butter, or ghee, etc., can be dangerous. Generally,

oil made from soybeans or peanuts is useful for the body provided that it is taken in limited quantities.

- **Salt:** Most patients are advised to reduce their salt intake. They are asked not to add table salt, eat foods prepared with yeasts or in very small quantities. Salt substitutes should be avoided because they are high in potassium.

- **Kinds of cereal:** rice and derived products such as flattened or poha rice, puffed rice, or kurmura can be eaten. To avoid taking a single type of cereal, we can vary by taking wheat, rice, poha, sorghum, semolina, and all the flours and cornflakes offered on the market. Barley, corn, and barja should be limited.

- **Seasoning sauces:** different sauces can be taken in prescribed amounts and varying to improve the acceptability of meals. As sauces are liquid, the amount of liquid consumed with it should be counted. If possible, use thick sauces rather than liquid ones. The proportion of sauces must be following the medical prescription.

- To reduce potassium in foods, it is important to soak them in hot water thrown away later after washing. Afterwards, they must be boiled and the additional water discarded. Thus, the ingredient is ready for the method of preparation of your choice. As an alternative to rice in sauces, you can take khichdi or dosha.

- **Plants:** Plants with a low potassium level can be taken without restriction. But plants rich in potassium must undergo the potassium extraction process before consumption. To improve the taste, lemon juice can be added.

- **Fruits:** fruits low in potassium like apples, papaya, and raspberries can be eaten once a day. On the day of the dialysis session, the patient can eat a piece of fruit. Fruit juices and water from the coconut should be avoided.

- **Milk and derived products:** 300 to 350ml of milk or its derivatives such as kheer (rice cake), ice cream, curdled milk, mattha can be consumed. Again, to avoid excess fluids, one should limit the amounts of these products.

- **Cold drinks:** Pepsi, Fanta, Frooti should be avoided. Do not take any fruit juice or water from the coconut.

- **Dried fruits:** Dried fruits, peanuts, sesame seeds, fresh or dry coconut should be avoided.

Chapter Seven:
7-Day Plan: What to Eat to Detoxify Your Kidneys Fast

Bad diets, environmental pollutants, and drug residues place a strain on the kidneys. What you need is time to regenerate the philtre organs. You should pay attention to how to get to know a way of life with it that is kidney-friendly and have healthy recipes.

Many think of the liver first when it comes to detoxification and relief. That is right. However, in terms of disposing of harmful substances, it is often overlooked that our kidneys also do amazing things and are vital. Using tiny philtres, the so-called nephrons, they clean over 1,000 litres of blood per day.

In doing so, urea, phosphates, toxins, and drug residues are filtered out, urine forms, and the pollutants are flushed out of the body. However, the philtre organs of about eight million Germans are constantly overloaded, and the function of the kidneys is already impaired. Our lifestyle with poor diet, obesity, high blood pressure, and diabetes is the primary cause.

You should keep this in mind when cleaning and detoxifying the kidneys.

Foods that contain a lot of these substances should therefore at least be reduced during the 7-day kidney detox. The ten most important rules are:

- Avoid sausage and red meat.

- No fast food, no ready meals, please prepare everything yourself as much as possible—then you will know what's in it.

- Eat lots of fresh vegetables and fruits.

- Pay attention to fibre every day, not only whole meal bread but also psyllium husks or flaxseed.

- Season only sparingly with salt, preferably with fresh herbs.

- Refrain from alcohol and coffee.

- Largely reduce fat and sugar.

- Drink around two litres of water a day. More is not good for kidney function unless you sweat a lot, then you should drink more to compensate for the loss of fluid. Important: Not in a few large portions, but a small glass now and then throughout the day. This cleanses the kidneys particularly well.

- Freshly squeezed lemon juice is deacidified (has an alkaline effect in the body due to its minerals) and can protect against kidney stones, as studies show. Drinking the juice of a lemon every day is therefore considered prevention for the kidneys, but also generally for detoxification.

- **Also important:** Set your kidney week as stress-free as possible and ensure relaxation. Stress is an often-underestimated "enemy" of the kidneys.

Kidneys Detox Day 1

- **Breakfast:** herbal tea to taste, whole meal bread with low-fat quark, seasoned with freshly ground caraway seeds, paprika, turmeric.

- **Lunch:** Carrot pasta with spring onions and pine nuts. To do this, cook the whole grain ribbon pasta until soft, sauté the carrots and onions in a little safflower oil during the cooking time, then roast the pine nuts and add them. Mix everything on a large platter, season with fresh herbs such as parsley, and pour a few ricotta dabs over the top.

- **Dinner:** oven vegetables. To do this, wash sweet potatoes, bell peppers, onions, garlic, potatoes, aubergines (choose according to your taste), cut into strips, and place on a tray greased with olive oil, bake at 200° C, season with fresh herbs such as rosemary. If that's too dry for you: Season skimmed yoghurt with garlic and fresh dill and use as a dip.

- **In between/snack:**

- Fruit.

- Whole grain pastries, such as sesame pretzel, without the salt crumble.

- Green vegetable smoothie, for example, with kohlrabi and cucumber, water.

- Juice of one freshly squeezed lemon, diluted with tap water.

Kidneys Clean Day 2

- **Breakfast:** muesli made from oat flakes, some flaxseed, berries, and low-fat yoghurt, herbal tea.

- **Lunch:** pasta salad with sun-dried tomatoes and oranges. To do this, cook pasta such as farfalle or penne al dente, chop the dried tomatoes, and fillet an orange. Serve the tomato strips and orange fillets with a little olive oil, chop the fresh parsley or chervil and season the dressing with it, add fine fruit vinegar to taste, mix with the pasta.

- **Dinner:** tomatoes and cucumbers with mozzarella, flavoured with high-quality olive oil and fresh basil, served with whole grain bread.

- **In between/snack:**

    - Fruit.

    - Whole grain pastries, such as sesame pretzel, without the salt crumble

    - Orange-red smoothie, for example, with berries, orange and carrot, water.

    - Juice of one freshly squeezed lemon, diluted with tap water.

Kidneys Clean Day 3

- **Breakfast:** Whole grain bread with cream cheese made from goat or sheep milk, seasoned with fresh herbs to taste, such as chives.

- **Lunch:** poultry steak with paprika vegetables (red, yellow, and green peppers, onions, some sour cream) and rice.

- **Dinner:** apple crumble. To do this, peel tart apples, cut into slices, and place in a lightly buttered baking dish. Drizzle with the juice of one lemon. From 100 grams of whole meal flour, a handful of oat flakes, 80 grams of brown sugar, and just as much butter, a pinch of cinnamon, knead a crumbly mass and sprinkle it over the apples, bake in the oven at 200° C.

- **In between / snack:**
  - Fruit.
  - Whole grain pastries, such as sesame pretzel, without the salt crumble.
  - Green vegetable smoothie, for example with banana, cucumber, green lettuce, rice milk.
  - Juice of one freshly squeezed lemon, diluted with tap water.

Kidneys Clean Day 4

- **Breakfast:** muesli with seasonal berries or apples, buckwheat flakes, oat milk.

- **Noon:** Italian bread salad. To do this, cut the ciabatta into slices, divide into bite-sized cubes, rub with a cut clove of garlic and moisten a little olive oil, briefly toast on a baking sheet in the oven. In the meantime, chop the tomatoes, cucumber, and onions for the salad and place in a large bowl. Prepare the vinaigrette from olive oil, balsamic vinegar, and lots of fresh herbs to taste, mix with the vegetables. Let the bread cool down briefly, fold into the salad and enjoy.

- **Dinner:** vegetable soup (minestrone). Prepare vegetable broth from vegetables to taste—beans, zucchini, carrots, fennel, celery—first sauté the vegetables in olive oil, then fill up with a little water; season with bay leaf, basil, and a pinch of salt (no more). Just before cooking, stir in a handful of soup noodles.

- **In between/snack:**

    - Fruit.

    - Whole grain pastries, such as sesame pretzel, without the salt crumble.

    - Smoothie red, roughly with seasonal berries and banana, water.

    - Juice of one freshly squeezed lemon, diluted with tap water.

Kidneys Clean Day 5

- **Breakfast:** scrambled eggs from two eggs, pour over a diced tomato, season with fresh herbs, with whole meal bread.

- **Lunch:** risotto with radicchio. To do this, sauté risotto rice in olive oil, add a finely diced onion and a clove of garlic, fry briefly, pour a little vegetable stock, and cook over low heat. In another pan, sauté the sliced radicchio in olive oil, add a little salt, add a dash of oat cream and add this vegetable mixture to the risotto, fold in slightly; season with fresh rosemary.

- **Evening:** Baked vegetable stew. To do this, put the finely chopped vegetables of your choice in an ovenproof casserole dish with a lid, such as beans, pumpkin, tomatoes, courgettes, peppers, onions, kohlrabi. Add a cup of water, season with a little salt but a lot of herbs, if you like, also some chilli, cover and cook at 180° C for about 30 minutes. Then pour the ricotta flakes over the casserole and enjoy with the whole-wheat baguette.

- **In between/snack:**

    - Fruit.

    - Whole grain pastries, such as sesame pretzel, without the salt crumble.

    - Green smoothie, for example, with lettuce, pineapple, cucumber, and water.

- Juice of one freshly squeezed lemon, diluted with tap water.

Kidneys Clean Day 6

- **Breakfast:** Muesli made from millet, seasonal fruit, and rice milk.

- **Noon:** Salmon Pasta with lemon and zucchini. To do this, sauté the salmon and zucchini in a little olive oil, add a little sour cream, season with fresh lemon juice and a little salt. Boil the pasta and mix both, grind the pepper over it.

- **Dinner:** sauté fried aubergines, aubergine slices, and onion slices in a little olive oil, flavour with lemon, add cherry tomatoes and capers to taste. Rice or whole grain baguettes go well with it.

- **In between/snack:**

    - Fruit.

    - Whole grain pastries, such as sesame pretzel, without the salt crumble.

    - Green vegetable smoothie, for example, with romaine lettuce, apple, and water.

    - Juice of one freshly squeezed lemon, diluted with tap water.

Kidneys Clean Day 7

- **Breakfast:** whole grain bread with herbal cream cheese.

- **Lunch:** Gnocchi with tomatoes. Make gnocchi yourself from 500-grams of floury, boiled potatoes, press through a sieve or mash, and knead with 125-grams of flour and an egg, season with a pinch of salt, and nutmeg. Shape the potato dough into rolls, cut small slices, press a fork on each piece, put in boiling water. When the gnocchi float up, they are done. Simply drizzle with a little liquid butter and flavour with fresh sage, or serve with a simple tomato sauce (fresh tomatoes, onion, garlic, a pinch of salt, a teaspoon of honey). Gnocchi is excellent for freezing, so simply make double the amount and store them in the freezer.

- **Dinner:** asparagus with green vinaigrette, peeled green or white asparagus, boil, drain, prepare vinaigrette with olive oil, balsamic vinegar, and fresh herbs as desired with whole meal baguette.

- **In between/snack:**
    - Fruit.
    - Whole grain pastries, such as sesame pretzel, without the salt crumble.
    - Red smoothie, for example with beetroot (cooked), apple, water.
    - Juice of one freshly squeezed lemon, diluted with tap water.

Myths and Facts about Kidney Disease

- **Myth:** All kidney disease is incurable

Reality: No, not at all. Kidney disease is curable if it is diagnosed early, and treatment is given immediately. Often the disease stops its progression or progresses very slowly.

- **Myth:** kidney failure can happen as soon as a kidney fails

Reality: No, kidney failure happens when it affects both kidneys. Often, there are no clinical manifestations with just one kidney, and the values of creatinine and urea are normal in the blood. But if both kidneys are affected, the body accumulates waste, and creatinine and urea in the blood increase, indicating kidney failure.

- **Myth:** In kidney disease, edema means kidney failure.

Reality: No. In some kidney diseases, edema is present while the kidney function is completely normal (e.g., nephrotic syndrome).

- **Myth:** In all patients with renal failure, edema is present.

Reality: No. Edema is present in the majority of patients with renal failure, but not all. Patients with advanced renal failure without edema are rare but exist. Indeed, the absence of edema does not rule out the possibility of renal failure.

- **Myth:** All kidney disease patients should drink plenty of water.

Reality: No. Reduced urinary excretion leads to significant edema in renal disease. It is, therefore, necessary to make a water restriction to maintain a good balance in some patients with certain kidney diseases. However, patients with kidney stones or urinary tract infections and normal kidney function should drink plenty of water.

- **Myth:** I'm fine, so I don't think I have kidney problems.

Reality: Most patients are asymptomatic (they have no symptoms) during the early stages of chronic kidney disease. Only the high biological values of creatinine and urea are the only key arguments at these stages.

- **Myth:** I feel great and better; I don't think I need treatment for my kidney problems yet.

Reality: Many patients with chronic kidney disease feel good with the right treatment and therefore stop their medications and diet. Interrupting medication and not following the regimen can be dangerous. They can lead to rapid deterioration of kidney function, requiring dialysis or transplantation in a much shorter time.

- **Myth:** Dialysis performed once in a patient becomes a permanent necessity.

Reality: No, the time on dialysis needed for a patient depends on the type of kidney failure.

Acute renal failure is temporary and reversible. Some patients require the temporary recourse to dialysis, but most often, following medical treatment combined with a few dialysis sessions, the kidney recovers its functions and completely. The delay in starting dialysis for fear that this need is permanent threatens the vital prognosis. Chronic kidney disease progresses irreversibly to kidney failure. At an advanced or terminal stage, the need for lifelong dialysis is essential.

- **Myth:** Dialysis cures kidney failure.

Reality: No, dialysis does not cure kidney failure, but it is an effective, life-saving treatment for patients with kidney failure by ridding their blood of toxic wastes and excess fluids and correcting electrolyte and acid-base disorders. Dialysis plays the role of the kidney that is no longer able to do its job. It allows patients to become asymptomatic and to be in good health despite their severe kidney failure.

- **Myth:** In kidney transplantation, men cannot give to women and vice versa; transplantation is not possible between the two sexes.

Reality: Men and women can donate to the opposite sex since the structure and functions of the kidney are the same in both.

- **Myth:** Kidney donation can affect the health and sexual function of the donor.

Reality: Kidney donation is completely harmless and safe and has no effect on the health of donors or their sexual functions. Donors live normally, get married, and have children.

- **Myth:** If you want a kidney transplant, you can buy it.

Reality: Selling or buying kidneys is a crime. A transplanted kidney from an unrelated living donor has a higher risk of rejection than a kidney from a related one.

- **Myth:** Now, my blood pressure has returned to normal and I no longer need high blood pressure treatment. I feel better when I don't take it so, why am I going to keep taking it?

Reality: Many hypertensive patients stop treatment if blood pressure becomes normal, especially since they no longer have symptoms or are better off without it. But uncontrolled high blood pressure is a silent killer that can lead to long-term complications like heart attacks, kidney failure, and stroke. So, to protect these noble organs of the body, it is essential to take your treatments regularly and to regularly measure your blood pressure even in the absence of symptoms and that you are in good health.

- **Myth:** Only men have kidneys in a pocket between the legs

Reality: In both men and women, the kidneys are located in the back and upper part of the abdomen, and they are the same size and function. What men have in a sac between their legs are reproductive organs or testes.

CPSIA information can be obtained
at www.ICGtesting.com
Printed in the USA
BVHW011509220221
600778BV00012B/1406